R
854
.U5
B3
198

WITHDRAWN

Date Due

NOV 1 1 '95			
DEC 1 4 1998			
DEC 0 7 2001			

BRODART, INC.   Cat. No. 23 233   Printed in U.S.A.

Springer Series on
Health Care and Society

Steven Jonas, M.D., *Series Editor*
Advisory Board:
H. David Banta, M.D.
Bonnie Bullough, R.N., Ph.D.
Kurt W. Deuschle, M.D.
Robert L. Kane, M.D.
Roger Meyer, M.D.
Ruth Roemer, J.D.

Volume 1
Quality Control of Ambulatory Care:
A Task for Health Departments
Steven Jonas

Volume 2
Community Medicine in the United Kingdom:
Medical Education and an Emerging Specialty within the Reorganized National Health Service
William S. Jordan, Jr.

Volume 3
Social Medicine:
The Advance of Organized Health Services in America
Milton I. Roemer

Volume 4
Patient Education:
An Inquiry into the State of the Art
Wendy D. Squyres, *Editor*

Volume 5
Toward Rational Technology in Medicine:
Considerations for Health Policy
H. David Banta, Clyde J. Behney, and Jane Sisk Willems

Volume 6
Staffing Primary Care in 1990:
Physician Replacement and Cost Savings
Jane Cassels Record, *Editor*

H. David Banta, M.D., M.P.H., is the manager of the health program in the Office of Technology Assessment (OTA), a research agency of the Congress of the United States. He has directed three studies for OTA concerning the evaluation of medical technology and now directs a research team doing studies on a number of health-related topics. Dr. Banta received his M.D. from Duke University in 1963, and was awarded an M.P.H. and an M.S. from Harvard University in 1968 and 1969. Previously, he was on the faculty of community medicine of the Mount Sinai School of Medicine in New York. His main professional activity involves carrying out and directing policy research related to technology and health. The relation of technology to society, in both industrialized and nonindustrialized nations, is his primary interest. His extensive contributions to the scientific literature have concerned health policy, medical technology, primary care, consumer participation, and medical education.

Clyde J. Behney, M.B.A., is a senior analyst in the health program of OTA. He has worked on the studies of saccharin, the CT scanner, and the efficacy and safety of medical technologies. During 1979 and 1980 he directed an assessment of the implications of cost-effectiveness analysis in health care. Before coming to OTA he worked in several agencies of the U.S. Department of Health, Education, and Welfare. He received a B.S. from Lehigh University in 1968 and an M.B.A. from the University of Maryland in 1972. He is interested in the relation of medical technology to social values.

Jane Sisk Willems, Ph.D., is a Veterans Administration Scholar resident at the National Center for Health Services Research. From 1976 to 1978 she worked at OTA where she helped direct studies on the CT scanner and on federal vaccine and immunization policies. During 1979 and 1980 she served on the advisory panel to the OTA study on cost-effectiveness analysis. She received a B.A. from Brown University in 1963, an M.A. from George Washington University in 1965, and, a Ph.D. in economics from McGill University in 1976. She is interested in the effect of organization on the delivery of medical care and, as a VA Scholar, is examining the use of technologies and the costs of care in different practice arrangements. She is also interested in the different activities through which the United States and other countries address similar issues of modern medical technology.

TOWARD RATIONAL TECHNOLOGY IN MEDICINE
Considerations for Health Policy

H. David Banta, M.D., M.P.H.
Clyde J. Behney, M.B.A.
Jane Sisk Willems, Ph.D.

Foreword by Senator Edward M. Kennedy

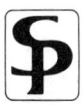

Springer Publishing Company
New York

*To Daniel Zwick
who taught us by example that
"bureaucrat"
can be an honorable word*

Copyright © 1981 by Springer Publishing Company, Inc.

All rights reserved

No part of this publication may be reproduced, stored in a retrieval system, or transmitted in any form or by any means, electronic, mechanical, photocopying, recording, or otherwise, without the prior permission of Springer Publishing Company, Inc.

Springer Publishing Company, Inc.
200 Park Avenue South
New York, New York 10003

81 82 83 84 / 10 9 8 7 6 5 4 3 2 1

Library of Congress Cataloging in Publication Data

Banta, H. David
  Toward rational technology in medicine.

  (Springer series on health care and society; v. 5)
  Bibliography: p.
  Includes index.
  1. Medical innovations—United States. 2. Medical policy—United States. 3. Medical care—United States.
I. Behney, Clyde J., joint author. II. Willems, Jane Sisk, joint author. III. Title. IV. Series. [DNLM:
1. Technology, Medical—United States. 2. Health policy—United States. W1 SP685S v.5 / WB 365 B219t]
R854.U5B36   362.1'068'2   80-27512
ISBN 0-8261-3200-6
ISBN 0-8261-3201-4 **(pbk.)**

Printed in the United States of America

Contents

Foreword by Senator Edward M. Kennedy vii

Preface xi

1. Medical Technology: Concepts and Concerns 1
2. Historical Perspective on Technology in Medicine 21
3. Research and Development 37
4. Adoption of Medical Technologies 53
5. Factors Affecting Use of Technology by Providers 75
6. Evaluation of Efficacy and Safety 93
7. Costs and Their Evaluation 123
8. Medical Technology and Social Values 137
9. Assuring the Quality of Medical Care 157
10. Selected Experience of Other Countries 173
11. Strategies for Improvement 189

Appendix A: Office of Technology Assessment—Health Program Reports 203

Appendix B: Glossary of Acronyms; Organization Chart (Department of Health and Human Services) 209

References/Additional Readings 213

Index 237

Foreword

Senator Edward M. Kennedy

Americans have an abiding faith that new knowledge can improve their lives. I share this belief. I am proud that our country has had the wisdom to invest generously over the last 30 years in biomedical and behavioral research aimed at the conquest of disease.

The result has been an unprecedented explosion of medical technologies for the prevention, diagnosis, and cure of disease. In most cases, these new technologies have had unquestioned benefit; they have ended or eased suffering and disability. Many lives have been saved. Many families have been given hope instead of grief and despair.

Yet we also must recognize that some of the new technologies have been rushed into widespread use before their safety and efficacy have been thoroughly tested and established. Several of the technologies seem to be overutilized and questions have been raised about the social and ethical impact of others. So now we must begin to balance the benefits, risks, costs, and social implications of each new technology. As the cost of medical care rises in a time of limited private and public resources, we must insist that resources be spent wisely and we must recognize that not every new or conceivable technology is necessarily an advance.

Problems with the development and application of new technology in general, and medical technology in particular, first came to the attention of Congress in the late 1960s and early 1970s. The difficulty of obtaining reliable information on the potential benefits and liabilities of technology led in 1972 to the passage of my legislation establishing the Office of Technology Assessment (OTA). In 1975, I proposed the development of a health program to the OTA Congressional Board; that program has become an indispensable means for understanding and anticipating the impact of technology on national health policy.

The role of OTA and its health program is only one of a number of developments that improve our ability to deal with new and existing technologies. The other major events include:

- The creation of Professional Standards Review Organizations (PSRO) to review and set standards for medical practice under the Medicare and Medicaid programs in the 1972 amendments to the Social Security Act;
- The coverage of treatment for end-stage renal disease in the same amendments;
- A new system for health planning, established in 1974, which provides that the National Council on Health Planning and Development must consider the implications of medical technology in its deliberations and recommendations;
- The establishment of the White House Office of Science and Technology Policy in 1976;
- The passage of the 1976 Medical Device Amendments requiring demonstrated efficacy and safety of medical devices.

As stated in the preface that follows, three studies considering the problems of medical technology were prepared some time ago at my request. These studies and a series of hearings I conducted in 1977 on technologies such as coronary bypass surgery, radical mastectomy, and gastric freezing provided dramatic evidence of the urgent need for a more thorough process for assessing medical technology. Efforts to that point had been fragmentary. Everyone was in the act, but the action was incomplete.

The need was now clear, and the Secretary of Health, Education, and Welfare, and the Surgeon General of the Public Health Service, established a Technology Management Task Force. It proposed a strategy by which the process of evaluating technologies would be nationally managed. The task force and OTA called for additional funds for research on medical technologies and for a mechanism to set research priorities. Their conclusions were convincing. A new agency was essential to assure the timely evaluation of new health technologies. In October 1978, Congress passed my legislation establishing the National Center for Health Care Technology. The creation of the center is a vital first step toward synthesizing and disseminating what is known about health care technologies.

However, evaluation itself cannot assure that worthwhile technologies will come rapidly into use. It cannot assure that technologies will be used appropriately. It cannot prevent ineffective or unsafe technologies from being used. It cannot control the rising costs of medical care. It cannot safeguard against the adverse social and ethical consequences of our scientific advances.

Foreword

The authors of this book, building on their reports at OTA, have outlined ways of dealing with the deeper challenges and dangers of medical technology. The message of their book is that the medical care system must be changed if we are to have rational technology in medicine; that our present fragmented system cannot assure the rational use of technology; and that our reimbursement system, especially, encourages irrational, wasteful, and sometimes harmful abuses and misuses of medical technology. The proposals I have made in the Congress over the past several years to develop a national health insurance plan have reflected a similar analysis of our problems. One of the major contributions of this book is that it shows why fundamental change in our reimbursement system is not only necessary, but inevitable.

This book discusses technology assessment lucidly and comprehensively. I recommend it not only to those who assess medical technologies but also to those who use our scientific advances and to those who rely on them.

"When, as is bound to happen sooner or later, the analysts get around to the technology of medicine itself, they will have to face the problem of measuring the relative cost and effectiveness of all the things that are done in the management of disease. They make their living at this kind of thing, and I wish them well, but I imagine they will have a bewildering time."

—*Lewis Thomas*

Preface

This book grows out of several reports prepared by the Office of Technology Assessment from 1975 to 1979. The Office of Technology Assessment (OTA) was created by statute in 1972 to provide Congress with "early indications of the probable beneficial and adverse impacts of applications of technology." The primary job of OTA is to perform assessments that will assist Congress. The act establishing OTA states that: ". . . it is essential that, to the fullest extent possible, the consequences of technological applications be anticipated, understood, and considered in determination of public policy on existing and emerging national problems." The members of Congress serving on the Technology Assessment Board, which controls OTA, voted in 1975 to establish a health program.

The reports that led to this book stemmed from a request by the Senate Committee on Labor and Public Welfare in a letter of February 6, 1975 signed by Senators Kennedy, Javits, and Williams. The request said, "A problem crossing the boundaries of both cost and quality concerns the use of new technology and procedures in health care. Before new drugs can be used, proof of efficacy and safety must be provided. However, no such legal requirement applies to new technologies and procedures. Recent studies in England have brought into question the efficacy of certain technologies although their use in both England as well as the U.S. is widespread and very costly. We request the OTA to establish a panel of outstanding individuals to examine current Federal policies and current medical practices to determine whether a reasonable amount of justification should be provided before costly new medical technologies and procedures are put into general use."

The first report based on this request examined the development and diffusion of medical technology and described different methods of "technology assessment." The second, performed at the additional request of the Senate Committee on Finance, examined a specific technology, the computed tomography (CT) scanner. Finally, the third examined the concepts of efficacy and safety and their evaluation, and suggested improvements in related public policy mechanisms. A subsequent OTA report analyzed Federal vaccine and immunization policies, using the pneumococcal vaccine as a case study. In September 1978, OTA began a study of the implications of cost-effectiveness analysis for the health care system. Although not completed when this book went to press, that study had considerable influence on our thinking.

All three authors were involved in the study of cost effectiveness. In addition, David Banta worked on the first three published reports; Clyde Behney worked primarily on efficacy and safety, but also on the CT scanner; and Jane Willems worked on the CT scanner and on vaccine and immunization policies. After leaving the OTA staff, Jane Willems worked on this book as a Veterans Administration Scholar resident at the National Center for Health Services Research.

Although these reports have been widely cited in the developing literature on medical technology and its evaluation, we decided to undertake this book to make the material more accessible. Further, each OTA report had only a limited scope, but we attempt here to give an overview of all important aspects of medical technology evaluation.

The book's title reflects our belief that the present system of providing medical care can be improved. We believe that application of the tools for scientific assessment of medical technologies can increase rationality in medicine as a whole. However, we recognize that preferences and goals are determined by many factors, of which rationality is only one. We believe in democracy and do not want a system controlled by technocrats or evaluators. Our goal is to see the system change in the direction of rationality. We do not believe that complete rationality is possible, nor would we want to live in a society that made rationality its highest goal.

In this book, we deal with traditional medical technology as normally used by physicians. We do not deal with broader social technologies, such as systems for delivering medical care. We also exclude mental health technologies and traditional technologies delivered by folk or lay healers. Nonetheless, we believe that the principles of evaluation described here are generally applicable to these technologies as well.

It is an axiom of ecology that everything is connected to everything else. We have obviously not discussed everything related to technology in this book. We are acutely aware of some of the omissions. In particular, we have not discussed the United States' or world economy in relation to medical technology. The medical sector is a service industry and a major employer worldwide. In the postindustrial society such services seem destined to grow not only as human goods or products but also as employers and as outlets for people's energy and creativity. We have not proposed a shrinkage of the investment in health care. Nor do we believe that our proposals necessarily imply such a shrinkage. It may or may not be rational social policy to

Preface

expand the health care sector of the economy. Our concern is that as a society we spend that money wisely, that we not hurt people in the process, and that we do not ignore significant opportunities to improve health and happiness in the mistaken belief that expensive medical technology can solve all of our ills. We have tried to develop these ideas in OTA reports.

OTA reports are developed and written by OTA staff. But in each report outside consultants are involved, and ordinarily an advisory panel assists in the development of the assessment. The health program has an overall advisory committee that has functioned actively since 1975, chaired by Dr. Frederick Robbins of Case Western Reserve University. Dr. Robbins' advice and support have been invaluable in the development of the health program and its work. The report on development of medical technology had an advisory panel chaired by Dr. Eugene Stead of Duke University, and the efficacy and safety study's panel was chaired by Dr. Lester Breslow of the UCLA School of Public Health. Both chairmen and their panels were of inestimable help. One member of both of those panels deserves special mention. Dr. Kenneth Warner of the University of Michigan has almost become a member of our staff and has worked with us on contract on our cost-effectiveness study. His ability to communicate economic concepts in plain English, as well as his knowledge and creativity, have made him an invaluable resource. The advisory panel to the cost-effectiveness study was chaired by Dr. John Hogness, the President of the Association for Academic Health Centers.

We are also grateful to staff of Congressional Committees and of individual Congressmen who have been particularly responsive to us. On the staff of the Health Subcommittee of the Senate Labor and Human Resources Committee, we have had fruitful working relationships with Stan Jones, David Blumenthal, and Bob Knouss. Stan Jones provided support for and interest in OTA during its early years. David Blumenthal deserves special credit for his staff work on the bill developed by Senator Kennedy to establish the National Center for Health Care Technology. On the staff of the Health Subcommittee of the Senate Committee on Finance, Jay Constantine deserves special recognition for his consistent and continuing commitment to assuring that medical services are efficacious and safe. We also have worked well with Jim Mongan, Bob Hoyer, and John Kern of that Subcommittee. On the staff of the House Interstate and Foreign Commerce Committee, George Hardy, Brian Biles, and Elliot Segal have been supportive and helpful. And on the House Ways and Means Committee, we have enjoyed our relationship with John "Mike" Holloman and Mary Nell Lehnhard.

Other OTA staff members made contributions to the reports and to our thinking. Joshua Sanes staffed the report on the development of medical technology and deserves special credit for his assistance in developing the list of questions presented in Chapter 8. Also, the material in Chapter 3 depends heavily on his work while at OTA. His knowledge of basic biological research, his writing ability, and his never-failing sense of humor made him a much-valued colleague. Carl Taylor, the first manager of the health program, was deeply committed to finding solutions to the problems of medical technology and continually challenged us to clarify both our thinking and our writing. Other staff members who made contributions include Dennis Andrulis, Larry Miike, Theresa Lucas, Michael Riddiough, Claudia Sanders, Page Gardner, and Kerry Kemp.

This book could not have been written without the help of several other individuals. First, Russell Peterson, Director of OTA from 1978 to 1979, encouraged us to undertake it. Second, the Assistant Director of OTA, Joyce Lashof, not only encouraged us, but read the entire book carefully and gave us many helpful comments and criticisms. She is of course not responsible for any errors. G. Barker-Benfield and Steve Jonas gave us constructive comments on a draft of Chapter 2. Louise Russell of the Brookings Institution is working with OTA as a consultant on the international papers summarized in Chapter 10 and made contributions to that chapter. Steve Thacker, Ken Warner, and Patricia Bauman read the entire manuscript and gave us many helpful comments. We also drew much support from our present colleagues at OTA. Particular thanks must be expressed to Ginny Cwalina for her administrative help and to Shirley Gayheart and Nancy Kenney for working long hours on the manuscript.

The book is organized to first provide the reader with a context for examining issues of medical technology. The first chapter introduces key concepts and concerns. The second chapter presents a historical perspective on these concerns. The next three chapters then deal with influences on technological change. Chapters 6 through 9 describe the effects of medical technology and methods for evaluating them. Chapter 10 examines the programs and experience of several other industrialized countries in trying to evaluate and control the effects of medical technologies. Finally, Chapter 11 suggests strategies for improving the present situation. Two appendices are provided. Appendix A contains brief descriptions of OTA Health Program reports. The second appendix includes an organization chart of the Department of Health and Human Services, as seen from the perspective of medical technology, and a glossary of acronyms used in the chart and in the rest of the book.

Though this book draws heavily upon our OTA experiences, any opinions are ours and do not represent official OTA policy.

1
Medical Technology: Concepts and Concerns

> The ability to face unprecedented situations by using the accumulated intellectual power of the race is mankind's most precious possession.
>
> Arthur E. Bestor

Technology

A society's technology inevitably changes that society. Technology has affected work patterns and roles, our diet, our sexual mores, our recreations, the concept of family, what we die of, and nearly every other aspect of life. Indeed, genetic technologies may change our very concept of life.

The subject of this book is medical technology, particularly in the context of national policy. It is concerned less with individual technologies than with the evaluation and appropriate use of medical technologies in general. As such it draws upon, and perhaps can contribute to, the discussions about the proper role in society of other types of technology.

The history of technology evokes both pride and despair. Its future breeds great hopes and terrible fears. Will the environment be saved or ruined by technology? Can medical technologies prevent or cure more cancers than are caused by technologies used in industry, agriculture, and the home? Are our energy and transportation problems susceptible to technological solutions? Is technology good, evil, or neutral? Is there a technological imperative in our culture that forces technology into our lives? Or, is it self-defeating to apply these terms to a tool or process? The answers to these and dozens of similar questions are crucial to society. There is a great deal of debate about possible answers, a great deal of searching. There is perhaps inevitable irony in a society that is built in large part on technology asking itself whether it can survive in the face of that technology. Ironic or not, the question is serious and certainly complicated. From all the noise generated by the technological debate, the one clear message is confusion. What should be done about technology and its power for good and ill?

This confusion over technology is partly an expression of the yet unresolved clash between the old order of unbridled optimism and a new wave of negativism. Technology the promise versus technology the peril; in the extreme, good versus evil, humanism versus mechanism. Neither view has to prevail, and neither should.

A healthy optimism regarding the potential of technology should be tempered by informed skepticism, not destroyed by it. Thus, this is not a doomsday book listing and predicting the dire consequences of technology run amok. It is, however, a critical look at society's ability to use its medical technologies wisely.

Definition of Technology

Technology is a term in search of a definition. It is important that the term be explicitly defined because it can take on such a broad range of meanings. Galbraith states that technology "means the systematic application of scientific or other organized knowledge to practical tasks" (Galbraith, 1977, p. 31). Elliott lists several views, including ". . . any tool or technique, any product or process, any physical equipment or method of doing or making by which human capability is extended" (Elliott and Elliott, 1976, p. 3). The wonderfully pessimistic Jacques Ellul is in substantial agreement with Lasswell's definition of "the ensemble of practices by which one uses available resources in order to achieve certain valued ends" (Ellul, 1964, p. 18). Ellul, however, implies that "practices," "resources," and "valued ends" must all be interpreted broadly.

What all these definitions, and dozens more, have in common is that they are broad, encompassing quite a large segment of human activity. One other aspect they share is that all were put forward or endorsed by people who spend a great deal of time and thought in the analysis of technology's meaning and effects. However, their general agreement on the essential nature of technology does not imply that that is how technology is viewed by most people. Another common reaction to the term technology is the creation of an image of physical objects such as machines or industrial plants. Mesthene states that:

> The research studies of the Harvard Program on Technology and Society reflect an operating assumption that the meaning of technology includes more

than machines. As most serious investigators have found, understanding is not advanced by concentrating single-mindedly on such narrowly drawn yet imprecise questions as "What are the social implications of computers, or lasers, or space technology"? Society and the influences of technology upon it are much too complex for such artificially limited approaches to be meaningful [Mesthene, 1977, p. 158].

He then goes on to critique the other extreme:

The opposite error, made by some, is to define technology too broadly by identifying it with rationality in the broadest sense. The term is then operationally meaningless and unable to support fruitful inquiry.

We have found it more useful to define technology as tools in a general sense, including machines, but also including linguistic and intellectual tools and contemporary analytic and mathematical techniques. That is, we define technology as the organization of knowledge for practical purposes. It is in this broader meaning that we can best see the extent and variety of the effects of technology on our institutions and values. Its pervasive influence on our very culture would be unintelligible if technology were understood as no more than hardware [Mesthene, 1977, pp. 158f].

The difficulties are obvious but, perhaps for our purposes, not terribly important. Some degree of imprecision may be inherent in the act of defining almost any concept that combines the abstract and the concrete. In this book, technology will simply be viewed as the purposeful application of organized knowledge. Although the derivation of the word indicates it should only be applied to a field of knowledge and implementation, we have followed accepted common usage in also applying it to specific techniques and procedures and to specific tools and machines.

Technology's Role in Society

The definition of technology encompasses both the simple and the complex. A windmill may be thought of as a technology, as may a multi-billion-dollar nuclear power plant. An organized system encompassing many technologies is itself a technology. Technology's role in society, then, can be said to be as old as the society in which it exists. Society feeds, clothes, and protects itself through its technologies, and it has always done so.

We still eat, go to work, make love, relax, and play games just as people have always done. Technologies have always played a role in these and most of society's other activities. How, then, has technology's role changed? Why has concern replaced optimism about that role? We can only suggest a few partial answers. First, although the essential function of a technology may not have changed, the power or intensity or scale of the technology needed to fulfill the function has often increased dramatically, accompanied by unforeseen consequences. Volumes of paper notebooks may have sufficed for our first national census but not for one of a population of over 200 million. Computers have the capacity to better accomplish this national project, but their necessarily greater power carries with it greater potential for unplanned side effects—for example, national data banks and decreased privacy. Similar examples could be cited in transportation, energy, communication, medicine, and so on.

Second, a technology not only serves a function but also tends to change that function. Automobiles were developed in response to an evolving societal desire for transportation. The effective function of personal transportation, however, was in turn altered by the availability of the automobile. Transporting an individual from a suburban home to an urban workplace is now regarded as one of the prime roles of the automobile, and that role not only was essentially unplanned but also has serious costs for the society (OTA, 1979a).

Third, concern about the role of technology also has increased, simply because of a greatly increased awareness of the implications of our extensive use of technologies. Interactive effects are increasingly recognized, and the relationship between transportation technologies and energy is an obvious example. Our knowledge of the unanticipated effects of technological applications also has grown. The dangers of x-rays serve as an example. So, too, do the long-term risks of exposure to asbestos or to constant and loud noises, to birth control pills, and to many other pharmaceuticals. With increased knowledge has come increased wariness about the possibility of other, as yet unidentified, unplanned effects.

Despite the growing concern over technology's role and effects, it remains an enormously pervasive aspect of our society. The 1970s were in fact the most technology-intensive decade in history, and the 1980s can probably be expected to follow suit.

That statement applies to most spheres of society and it certainly is applicable in medicine and health care.

Medical Technology

Extending the definition given above for technology to medical technology yields "application of organized knowledge for health-related purposes." This definition, though accurate, is too global for policymaking. The Office of Technology Assessment has found it useful to define medical technology as

> The drugs, devices, and medical and surgical procedures used in medical care, and the organizational and supportive systems within which such care is provided [OTA, 1978a].

Medical technologies are of many different types and serve a variety of functions. Nonetheless, they can be classified into sets. Schemes of classification can help in evaluating a particular technology and in judging new technologies on the basis of previous experience or evaluation.

A useful system for classifying medical technologies distinguishes these technologies according to two dimensions—medical purpose and physical nature. Each of these two dimensions can be broken down further as follows.

Medical purpose: (1) A *diagnostic* technology helps in determining what disease processes occur in a patient; (2) A *preventive* technology protects an individual from disease; (3) A *therapeutic* or *rehabilitative* technology relieves an individual from disease and its effects (therapeutic technologies can be further divided into those few technologies that cure disease and the many technologies that give symptomatic relief but do not alter the underlying disease process); (4) An *organizational* or *administrative* technology is used in management and administration to ensure that health care is delivered as effectively as possible; and (5) A *supportive* technology is used to provide patients, especially those in hospitals, with needed services (e.g., hospital beds and food services).

Physical nature: (1) A *drug* is any chemical or biological substance that may be applied to, ingested by, or injected into humans in order to prevent, treat, or diagnose disease or other medical conditions; (2) A *device* is any physical item, excluding drugs, used in medical care, and may range from a machine requiring large capital investment to a small instrument or implement; and (3) A *procedure* is a combination, often quite complex, of provider skills or abilities with drugs, devices, or both.

Drugs and devices are products; procedures, on the other hand, use a product or products according to the knowledge or skills of a medical care provider. In some cases, the drugs or devices involved are not predominant factors in a procedure. Instead, the technique of the provider performing the procedure is most import;ant. A surgical procedure, for example, involves the use of scalpels, clamps, and drugs against infection; the key to the procedure, however, is the surgeon's actions.

Changing Technology of Medicine

The technology available to the medical practitioner has changed remarkably in the past several decades. Just since 1940 a broad array of medical interventions has entered practice, including antibiotics; antihypertensive drugs; oral diuretics, oral contraceptives, psychopharmaceuticals; corticosteroids; polio, measles, mumps, and rubella vaccines; cardiovascular and open-heart surgery; genetic screening and amniocentesis; automated clinical laboratories; renal dialysis; and cardiac pacemakers (American Biology Council, 1972). However, essentially all of these remarkable advances entered practice before 1965. Although several dramatic advances, such as the CT scanner, have come into use since that time, the major change in the technology of medicine has been one of extent of diffusion and intensity of use.

Empirically Developed Technology

This book is largely concerned with scientific medicine—that is, medical technology that has resulted from science or scientific thought. The place of empirically developed technologies in the history of medicine is not clear. Histories have focused on the role of prominent medical scientists, especially physicians, and have paid little attention to other healers and lay people. Little has been written on techniques developed outside the formal system of medical care, even on those that were eventually incorporated into the system. Nonetheless, a complete history should cover such techniques, and some of that history is now being written. For example, healers of women are now receiving some attention: "Female lay healers did not have a rational theory of disease causation and therapy . . . but then they did not make any claims to 'book larnin.' What they did have was experience—experience which had been discussed and revised for generations" (Ehrenreich and English, 1979, p. 43). Indeed, medical orthodoxy has often prevented worthwhile technologies from being incorporated into health care. For example, ergot was used by midwives to contract the uterus at least as early as the sixteenth century, but it was not generally accepted by physicians until 1808 (Dowling, 1970, p. 15). Obstetrics unquestionably has profited much from techniques developed by lay midwives and, surely, similar points could be made for much of medicine.

To some degree, resistance to incorporating nontraditional medical techniques is understandable. Many lay remedies or procedures are probably not efficacious and safe. Some have their roots in superstition. On the other hand, much the same thing could be said about mainstream medical technologies. The crucial issues here are that (1) simply because a technology has been developed empirically by nonphysicians it should not automatically be discounted, and (2) *all* forms of technology can and should be evaluated for their effects and should not be accepted at face value.

The Process of Technological Change

The use of new technology by a consumer can be viewed as the culmination of a long sequence of activities (Hetman, 1973, p. 64). First, theoretical research and the sum of previous experience form a background or conceptual base. Then basic empirical research provides a framework of knowledge about the mechanisms involved in natural processes, discovers points in those processes that are susceptible to technological intervention, and suggests strategies for technological development. Applied or mission-oriented research is subsequently directed to applying this basic knowledge to a practical purpose and to demonstrating the feasibility of the proposed technology.

Once feasibility is determined, engineers and entrepreneurs and developers, usually in the private sector, develop implementation programs. For devices, the transfer of technology from the laboratory to the marketplace involves the construction of prototypes. Once the manufactured item is ready, its effectiveness and efficiency can be assessed realistically in industrial laboratories, in field tests, or in consultation with potential users. Drugs are often subjected to clinical trials at this point. Surgical procedures are more likely to be incorporated into practice by a practitioner who modifies an existing technique. The technology is then marketed and, if all goes well, adopted by the appropriate consumers, be they manufacturers or industries, public groups or institutions, or private individuals. The diffusion or incorporation of a technology into practice includes its adoption by potential users and its subsequent extent and pattern of use. Obsolescence or rejection of the technology is also a potential part of the process.

The development process of the cardiac pacemaker, shown in Figure 1-1, followed this sequence. Developing the pacemaker required the knowledge of anatomy, physiology, and pathophysiology that had accumulated over hundreds of years. Also required were advances in nonmedical fields, such as solid state physics and electrical engineering. Use of the pacemaker involves several devices plus surgery and drugs for implantation.

The development, diffusion, and use of medical technologies have been described as including at least seven steps (President's Biomedical Research Panel, 1976):

Figure 1-1.
Development of the Cardiac Pacemaker.

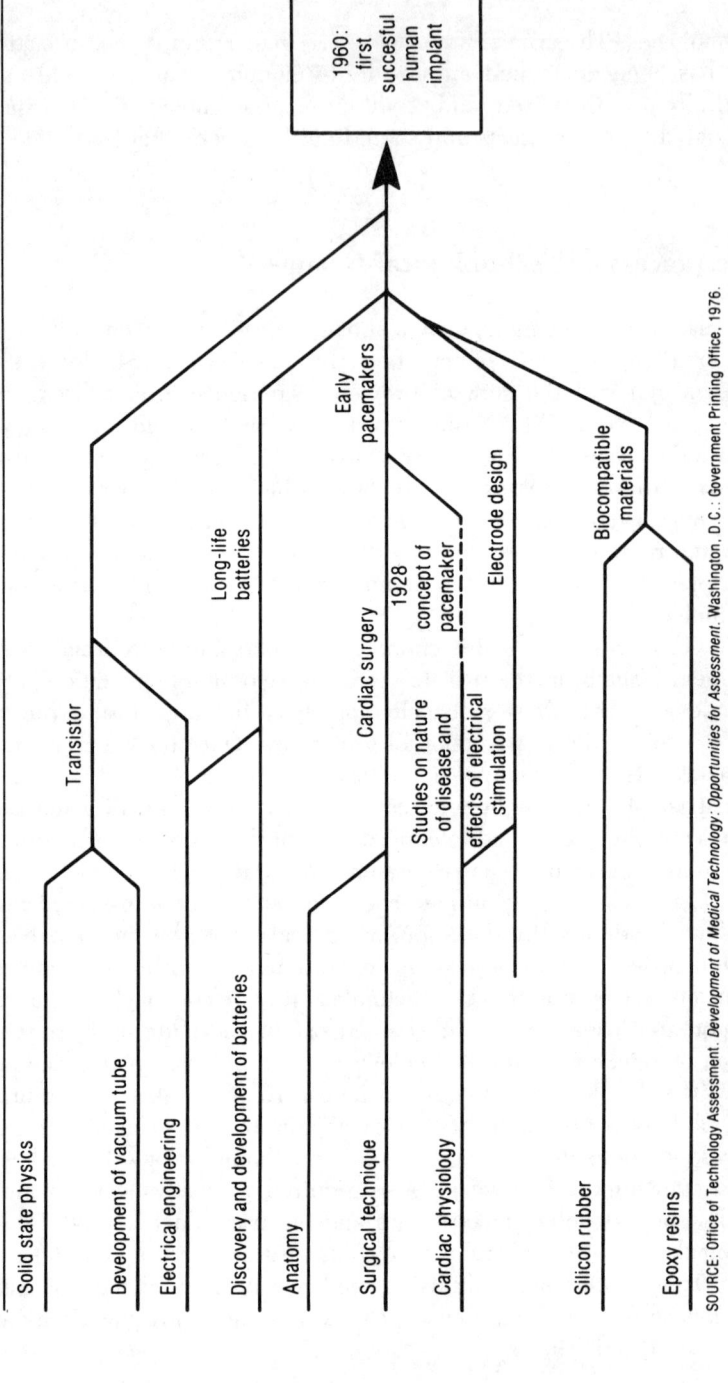

SOURCE: Office of Technology Assessment. *Development of Medical Technology: Opportunities for Assessment*. Washington, D.C.: Government Printing Office, 1976.

1. Discovery, through research, of new knowledge, and relation of this knowledge to the existing knowledge base;
2. Translation of new knowledge, through applied research, into new technology, and development of strategy for moving the technology into the health care system;
3. Evaluation of the safety and efficacy of new technology through such means as controlled clinical trials;
4. Development and operation of demonstration and control programs to demonstrate feasibility for widespread use;
5. Diffusion of the new technology, beginning with the trials and demonstrations, and continuing through a process of increasing acceptance into medical practice;
6. Education of the professional and lay communities in use of the new technology;
7. Skillful and balanced application of the new development to the population.

These steps are shown in Figure 1–2. (The bottom left-hand portion of the figure corresponds to the cardiac pacemaker example in Figure 1–1.)

This seven-step sequence offers a logical model for understanding the development process. The model suggests that it is often possible to identify and evaluate the effects of medical innovation prior to its widespread diffusion. But medical technologies, like others, emerge from a process that is far less systematic and certainly less linear than that which this model depicts. Despite its deficiencies, this scheme is used for convenience in this book.

The stage of development of a particular medical technology has a number of implications. For example, policies toward a new technology that is not yet in widespread use and those toward an older technology of questionable benefit that is widely used should be quite different. The National Council on Health Care Technology has defined three main stages in the life of a medical technology: emerging, new, and established. An emerging technology is in the applied research stage, either before or immediately after clinical testing. A new technology is one that is past the stage of clinical trials but not yet in widespread use. An established technology is one that is considered by providers to be a standard approach to a particular illness or disease condition and has diffused into general use. This scheme does not include a stage that should not be forgotten: obsolete, outmoded, or abandoned. The stage of development of a technology has important implications for its evaluation. For example, it may be difficult to evaluate a technology in widespread use because of ethical considerations, whereas such considerations are likely to be less of a problem with emerging technologies.

The length of time between the conception of an idea or innovation

Figure 1-2.
A Scheme for Development and Diffusion of Medical Technologies.

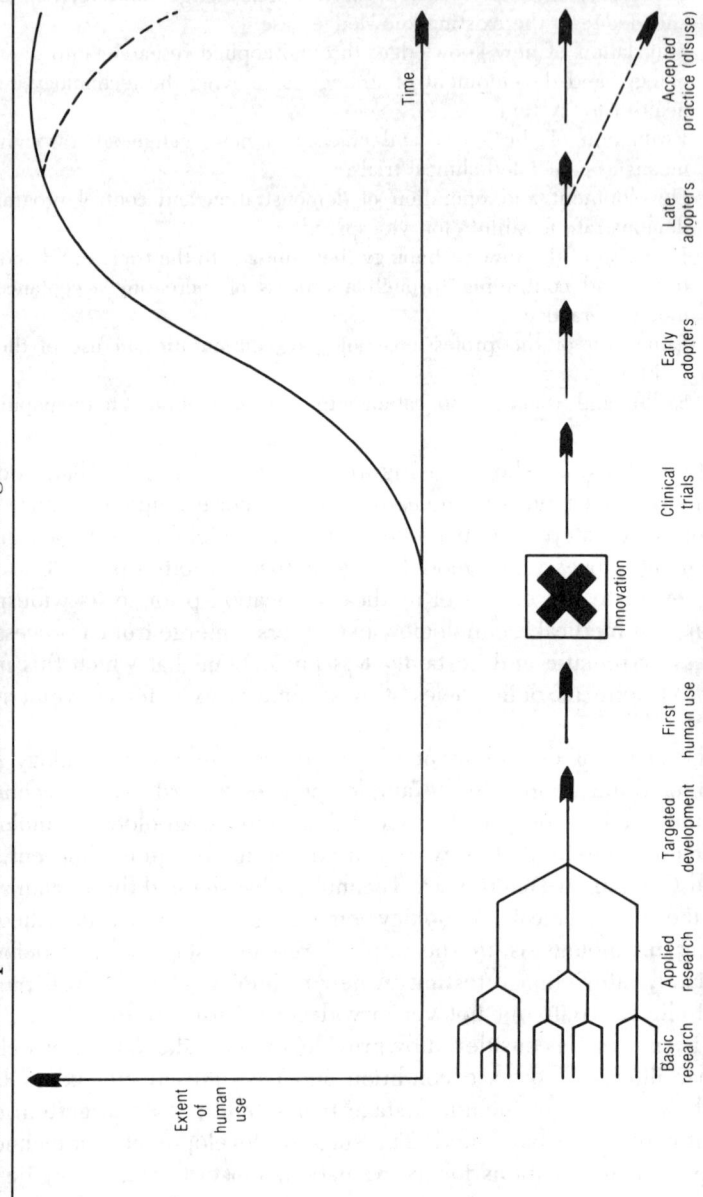

SOURCE: Office of Technology Assessment. *Development of Medical Technology: Opportunities for Assessment.* Washington, D.C.: Government Printing Office, 1976.

and the introduction into practice of the resultant technology—the so-called "bench to bedside lag"—has been debated for the last decade or so. There are, inevitably, lags. The lag should be neither too short nor too long. If too short, it may be that the technology was not completely developed or tested before it was introduced. If too long, patients who might benefit might be needlessly deprived of appropriate therapy. A number of investigators have studied the reasons for lags (Comroe and Dripps, 1976; Batelle, 1973; Batelle Columbus Laboratories, 1976). In most cases studied, reasons for long lags were limitations of knowledge or lack of supporting technology. Apparent lags can also result from delayed adoption of available techniques. Studies of the quality of medical care indicate that the most appropriate diagnostic or therapeutic procedures are often not used in clinical practice. One cause for lags pointed out by Comroe and Dripps (1976) and Batelle (1973) is a failure of communication: loss and subsequent rediscovery of important ideas, resistance to innovation by uninformed physicians, or academic skepticism to challenging new ideas. On the other hand, there are great social, economic, and human costs attached to prematurely accepting technology. Thus, attempts to understand and rationalize the development process must take account both of the possibility that some medical technologies are delayed in their development and the certainty that other technologies are diffused prematurely, before they are completely developed.

Concerns About Medical Technology

The concerns about the effects of medical technologies parallel those in other areas of technology: How can we identify the appropriate role of the technologies in question? And how can we assure that they will be put to that most appropriate use? For medical technologies, appropriate use depends on such factors as the health benefits and risks of the technologies, their financial effects, and their effects on social systems and values (Banta et al., 1979).

Benefits of Medical Technology

In many instances knowledge about disease has made it possible to develop effective methods of control—that is, technology. In some cases, this knowledge has been the result of epidemiological research, as when John Snow recognized patterns of cholera in London, resulting from ingestion of water from the Broad Street pump, and removed the handle of the pump as a disease preventive (MacMahon, 1960, pp. 154–155). Other preventive measures, such as vaccines, have resulted in part from knowledge of the structure of microorganisms; and many diagnostic and curative technologies have resulted from biomedical research, as well as research in such areas as engineering and physics.

These successes are most clearly seen in the case of infectious diseases. Vaccines have been developed for many of them. In other cases, antibiotics have made treatment and cure possible. Bennett has listed the following lethal and dangerous infectious diseases that medical technology can now control effectively: epidemic meningitis, infantile diarrhea, epidemic typhus, trachoma, scarlet fever, cholera, yellow fever, bacterial endocarditis, typhoid fever, leprosy, syphilis, gonorrhea, lobar pneumonia, malaria, measles, rubella, whooping cough, diphtheria, smallpox, tetanus, puerperal sepsis, and neonatal infection (Bennett, 1977). Figure 1-3 shows that in 1900 the leading causes of death were influenza and pneumonia, tuberculosis, gastritis, diseases of the heart, vascular lesions affecting the central nervous system, accidents, chronic nephritis, malignant neoplasms, diseases of early infancy, and diphtheria. Although six of these remain in the top ten causes of death in 1967 statistics, their relative importance has changed, so that the chronic diseases now predominate Mushkin (1979, p. 24) has reviewed studies of the costs and benefits of biomedical research, and finds some dramatic successes.

Many chronic diseases have also become controllable. Some examples are pellagra, rickets, scurvy, erythroblastosis fetalis, Addison's disease, juvenile diabetes, and certain types of cancer (Bennett, 1977). However, many chronic diseases do not have effective preventive and treatment measures. Large investments in biomedical research, high public expectations, and generous reimbursement systems have all helped to foster a kind of technology in these cases, which Thomas has called "halfway technology" (1974, p. 34). Such technologies are attempts to compensate for the incapacitating effects of certain diseases whose course one is unable to do much about. "It is a technology designed to make up for disease, or to postpone death." Thomas cites transplantations of hearts, kidneys, livers, and other organs, and the equally spectacular artificial organs. These measures address those diseases for which no definitive technology is available: stroke, heart attack, congestive heart failure, most forms of cancer, atherosclerosis, cirrhosis of the liver, emphysema, glomerulonephritis, pyelonephritis, osteoarthritis, asthma, multiple sclerosis, senility, schizophrenia, depression, mental retardation, muscular dystrophy, cystic fibrosis, and so forth (Bennett, 1977). It is not true that medicine has nothing to offer for these diseases. Rather, what it has to offer is often caring for the person rather

Figure 1–3.
Percent of All Deaths, by Specified Causes of Death* (U.S.A., 1900** and 1974).

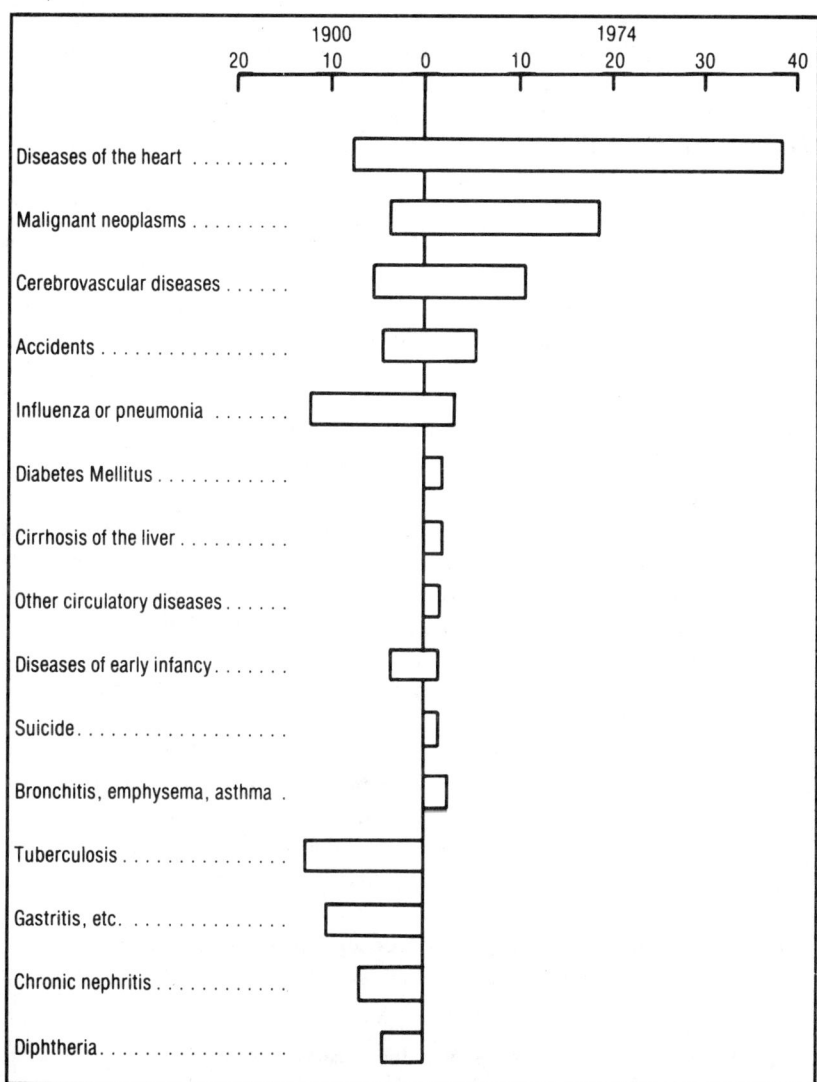

*10 leading causes of death in 1900 and 1974, with the latter arranged in descending order of importance.
**Death registration states only.
SOURCES: (1) For 1900: U.S. National Office of Vital Statistics. *Vital Statistics of the United States, 1950, Vol.1*, Washington, D.C., 1950, table 2.26, p. 170.
(2) For 1974: U.S. Department of Health, Education, and Welfare. Public Health Service, National Center for Health Statistics. *Monthly Vital Statistics Report*, Vol. 23, no.13, May 1975, table C, p. 3.

This figure is reprinted by permission of the University of Michigan. It appeared as chart B-5, *Medical Care Chartbook*, sixth edition, 1976.

than curing the disease. The result may be increased comfort or mobility, relief of pain, and reduced anxiety. These technologies often lack dramatic benefit, and they are often very expensive (Rosenthal, 1979).

From the above discussion it is clear that medical technologies have helped provide effective care to millions of people. They indisputedly provide dramatic benefits in some cases and are of some benefit in many others. How much benefit is gained, and—critically—under what circumstances, however, remains relatively unknown. Concerns have been raised about the benefits of a great many modern technologies; for example, electronic fetal monitoring (Banta and Thacker, 1979a), other obstetric practices (Chalmers and Richards, 1977), respiratory therapy (Barach and Segal, 1975), and oral drugs for diabetes (Knatterud et al., 1971; Chalmers, 1975). Chapter 3 describes in more detail the lack of knowledge about the efficacy (benefit) of medical technologies.

McKeown has approached the question of the importance of medical technology historically (1976). He describes the vast improvement in health during the past three centuries, and concludes that nutrition and the physical environment have been much more important for the prevention of sickness and death than have personal health care services. Death rates in England and Wales fell from about 22 per 1000 in 1841 to about 6 per 1000 in 1971. He shows that 92 percent of the fall between 1848 and 1901, and 73 percent from 1901 to 1971, is due to reduction in the number of deaths from infectious diseases. The greatest contributor to this fall was tuberculosis, which he analyzes in depth.

Figure 1-4 shows annual death rates due to respiratory tuberculosis beginning in 1838. The death rate has fallen steadily, although chemotherapy for tuberculosis did not begin until 1948. Figure 1–5 shows the period 1921 to 1970 in more detail, and it can be seen that after 1948 there is a change in the trend in the death rate, indicating an effect of therapy.

McKeown (1976) also examines other disease conditions. After tuberculosis, the greatest causes of mortality have been bronchitis, pneumonia, and influenza. The death rate for these conditions has been little affected by the introduction of antibiotics. Based on these and other observations, McKeown draws the following conclusions (pp. 93–94):

1. Improvement in nutrition was the earliest, and, over the whole period since about 1700, the most important influence.
2. Hygienic measures were responsible for at least a fifth of the reduction of the death-rate between the mid nineteenth century and today. . . .
3. With the exception of vaccination against smallpox, whose contribution was small, the influence of immunization and therapy on the death-rate was delayed until the twentieth century, and had little effect on national mortal-

Figure 1-4.
Respiratory Tuberculosis: Mean Annual Death Rates (Standardized to 1901 Population): England and Wales.

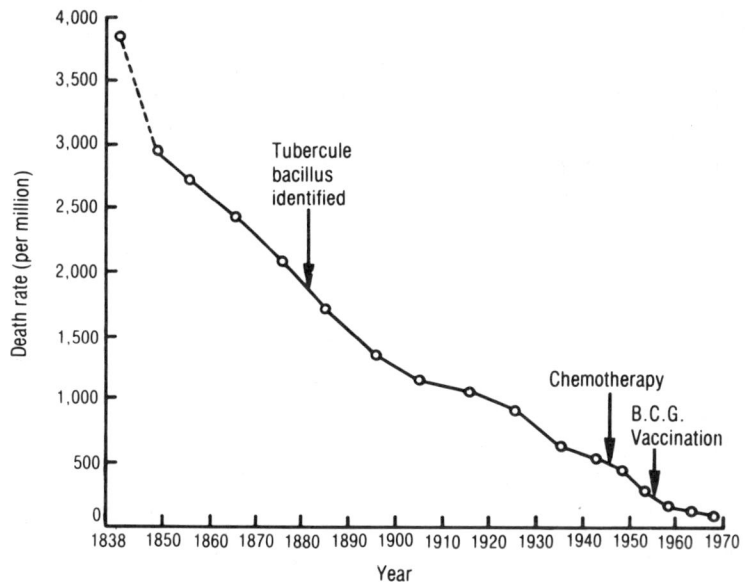

SOURCE: McKeown, T. *The Role of Medicine: Dream, Mirage or Nemesis?* London: Nuffield Provincial Hospitals Trust, 1976. Redrawn by OTA. Used by permission.

ity trends before the introduction of sulphonamides in 1935. Since that time it has not been the only, or probably the most important influence.
4. The change in reproductive practice which led to the decline of the birthrate was also very signigicant. . . .

He states in summary, "We have overestimated the effectiveness of many procedures and services in current use, and indeed most have been adopted without adequate evaluation" (pp. 118–119). Note that this does not imply that technology has been unimportant in the improvement in death rates, but rather that it has been environmental and other technologies more than clinical medical technologies that have brought the impact.

Mushkin has criticized this approach as putting too much emphasis on one biomedical advance. Using a different approach, a multivariant analysis of the products of research and of mortality rates, she finds that biomedical advances accounted for 30 to 40 percent of the reduction in deaths during the period 1900 to 1975.

Figure 1-5.
Respiratory Tuberculosis: Annual Death Rates of Males: England and Wales.

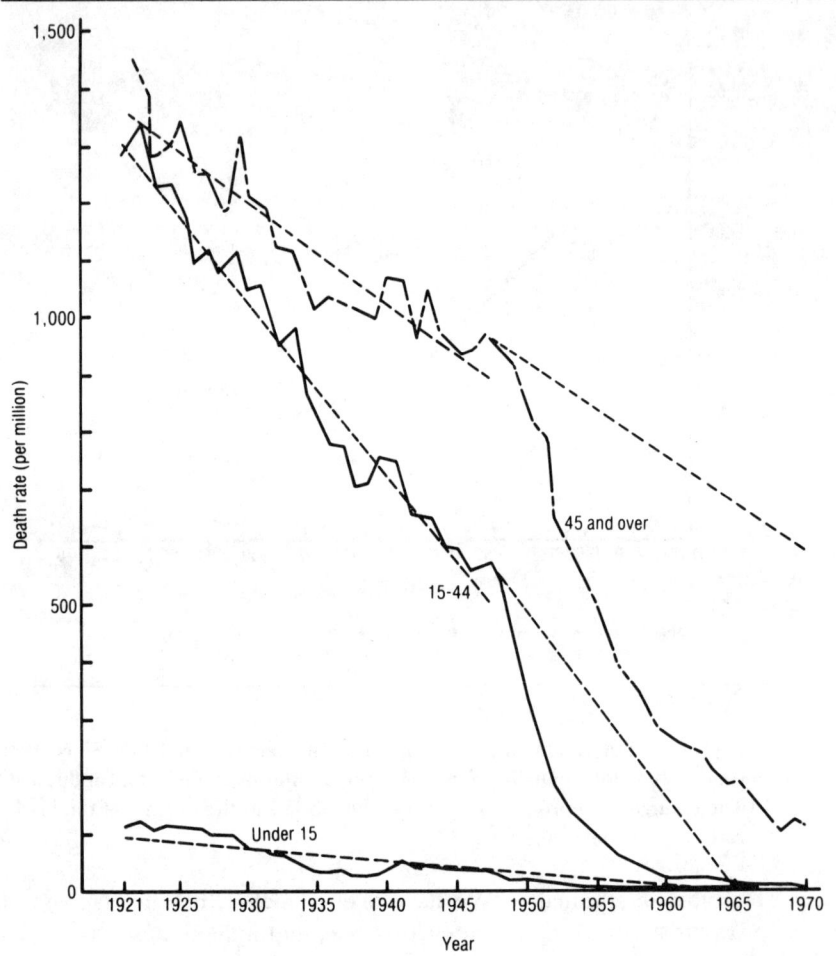

SOURCE: McKeown, T. *The Role of Medicine: Dream, Mirage or Nemesis?* London: Nuffield Provincial Hospitals Trust, 1976. Redrawn by OTA. Used by permission.

It should also be noted that medical care is more than just technology. Diseases occur in people, who have fears and anxieties. Therefore, much of medical practice is taken up with psychological problems and physical complaints that do not require the application of technology, but do require a concerned health care provider to provide reassurance and advice. Furthermore, there is no effective therapy for many chronic conditions. "Traditionally, medical care has served as much to relieve pain and anxiety and system function as it has to effect cures. Medical care is a highly personalized service with both physical and psychologic elements; these are highly related in the consumer's motivation to seek service and in the physician's ability to achieve cooperation by his advice and to change behavior to be conductive to health" (Sun Valley Forum, 1972).

Risks of Medical Technology

All technology has risks. In many cases, these are small, unquantifiable risks, and perhaps can be ignored if benefits are significant. However, the risks of many medical technologies are significant and have not been taken fully into account.

Drug risks have perhaps been more publicized than any other. It was the effect of thalidomide on the unborn child that led to the 1962 amendments to the Food, Drug, and Cosmetic Act (Dowling, 1970, p. 201). A more recent dramatic example of a side effect is the vaginal cancer now appearing in young women whose mothers were given estrogens during pregnancy (Lambert, 1978, p. 94). Although these are dramatic, the more typical risk is probably similar to that which accompanies drug treatment for hypertension: dizziness, impotence, and general tiredness (OTA, 1978a, p. 49). Although not life-threatening, these side effects are annoying enough to keep many patients from taking medication faithfully.

The risks of major surgery are obvious. For example, the risks of coronary bypass surgery include a hospital mortality of about 4 percent and myocardial infarction during surgery in about 7 percent of patients (Avery et al., 1976, pp. 429–431). Morbidity from complications such as thrombophlebitis (clots in the leg veins) is common with any major surgical procedure. Estimates of deaths from tonsillectomy range as high as 300 per year in the United States (OTA, 1978a, p. 44).

In many cases the risks are not so obvious. For example, screening for breast cancer by mammography, a special x-ray examination, exposes the breast to x-rays, which themselves cause cancer. The dose from the procedure can be below one rad, which has not been proved to be associated with a measurable risk. The risk of such x-rays may be finite, but this has not been quantified (OTA, 1978a, p. 33; BEIR Report, 1972).

Since essentially all technology is associated with risk, it is necessary to consider benefit in relation to risk for any given technology.

Financial Costs of Medical Technology

Medical technology has become a policy issue primarily because of the rapidly rising expenditures on medical care. Health expenditures as a percentage of the Gross National Product have doubled from 4.5 percent in 1950 to 9.1 percent in 1978 (National Center for Health Statistics, 1980, p. 244). These changes are primarily attributable to changes in the size, complexity, and cost of the service package provided by hospital or physician, and are not due to increased utilization of services (Hanft et al., 1978). The price of a semiprivate hospital room more than tripled from 1965 to 1975, and physician fees nearly doubled over this 10-year period.

These dramatic increases have led to a search for the culprit (Altman and Blendon, 1979). The profusion of costly medical equipment is an obvious contributor to rising expenditures, and indeed Federal officials have concluded: "the long-term cumulative effect of adopting new health care technology is a major cause of the large yearly increases in national health expenditures" (Gaus and Cooper, 1978). Various attempts have been made to quantify the contribution of technology to these increases. These will be described in detail in Chapter 4. It does appear that technology accounts for up to 50 percent of the increase in the cost of hospital care over the last decade. However, analyses have not shown clearly what type of technology is most responsible for the rising costs. "Are the increases mostly small ticket items, such as tests and procedures, or are they big ticket purchases, such as open heart surgical units and intensive care facilities. Also, we cannot say what proportion of the increase was the result of technological advances or other factors, such as billing equipment" (Altman and Wallack, 1979). The work of Scitovsky and McCall (1976) documents a rise in the cost of treating a number of conditions over time, and shows that the cost rise resulted from more diagnostic and therapeutic procedures. For example, the average number of diagnostic tests for a perforated appendix rose from 5.3 in 1951 to 31.0 in 1971. This work is suggestive, but needs to be replicated and extended.

The contribution of a number of discrete technologies to rising costs has been analyzed. Although this work does not indicate which are the most important causes of the rise, it does have credibility in documenting that technology does cause a rise in costs. For example, intensive care alone has been found to account for approximately 15 percent of 1975 hospital costs (Russell, 1979). The costs of CT scanning are more than $500 million a year (Banta, 1980a). The cost of renal dialysis is nearing $1 billion a year (Rettig, 1979c). The costs of diagnosis appear to be increasing rapidly, with a cost of clinical laboratory services between $15 and $20 billion a year and a cost of x-rays of about $5 billion a year (OTA, 1976).

Thus, there seems little doubt that medical technology is a significant factor in the rising cost of medical care; hence there is pressure to scrutinize its value.

Social Impacts of Medical Technology

The effects of medical technologies on health (benefits and risks) and on costs are usually the most direct and obvious implications of their use. However, some medical technologies have social implications that may be at least as important as those more direct effects. For example, who can deny that the birth control pill and other contraceptive technologies have had enormous social impact? The changes in our society's values and institutions that have occurred in whole or in part because of birth control techniques include altered sexual mores and a changing role for women in society (McConnell, 1974).

Renal dialysis is another example. Questions have been raised about: Who shall live? (Whom shall we dialyze if we can't dialyze everyone in need? How do we decide?) Who will pay? (Most renal dialysis is now covered by a special program of Medicare.) This is more than a question of finances because it raises issues of individual and social responsibility, equity, and whether there is a right to life and health (Fox and Swazey, 1974, 1979). What is the impact on the quality of life for those on dialysis three times a week for the rest of their lives?

Procedures such as amniocentesis (testing for chromosomal abnormalities and biochemical defects in the fetus) raise questions about manipulating society's gene pool, about increased abortions, about societal sex ratios, and others. The artificial heart has overpowering ethical, economic, and psychiatric implications (OTA, 1976; National Heart and Lung Institute, 1973).

The use of medical technologies can affect: (1) ethics and morals, changing or challenging our fundamental values or beliefs; (2) the legal and political system, pertaining to allocating scarce resources, defining death and life, informed consent, and so on; and (3) the economic system, going beyond issues of the cost of health care by affecting such factors as employment, productivity, and the necessity for and size of income maintenance programs. In fact, medical technologies, dealing as they do with health, which is a socially defined concept, can affect nearly every aspect of society and its institutions (Illich, 1976).

Not all or even most medical technologies have such significant social implications. The importance of this type of implication, however, lies not in how frequently it may occur, but in the degree of social upheaval that may be caused. The aggregate effect of the many new technologies of medicine is itself important. Also, these types of effects are of concern because of the subtlety of their occurrence; they are often very difficult to anticipate or to identify.

Summary of Federal Reactions to These Concerns

The United States has a number of government structures that deal with different stages of medical technology development and use. However, we do not feel that these programs deal with the problem adequately. Although a substantial amount of medical care is financed by public funds, the system remains largely in private hands. One of the most highly respected of our public bodies is the National Institutes of Health (NIH), the major source of funds for biomedical research and technology development. However, the NIH does not systematically carry out evaluations of its products. Further, there has been no statutory mandate to assure the appropriate evaluation of the entire range of medical technologies, although 1978 legislation did establish a new agency for that purpose.

Because of concerns about quality and the rising cost of medical care, a number of programs have been developed to influence diffusion and use of medical technologies. The most effective of these is probably the Food and Drug Administration, which requires proof of safety and efficacy before drugs and devices can be marketed in the United States. However, FDA has little control over drugs and devices once they are marketed, and such technologies are frequently overused and used inappropriately. Since 1974, the United States has had a national health planning program, one of whose tasks is to control the cost of medical care through the control of capital expenditures. Finally, since 1972, physician-controlled organizations, the Professional Standards Review Organizations (PSROs), have been developed to review services provided under Federal reimbursement programs to assure appropriate medical care.

All of these regulatory programs are hampered by lack of information about the efficacy and safety (the benefits and risks) of medical technologies, especially their appropriate conditions of use. Analytic tools are available to provide better data, but they have been little applied. Too little is known about usual medical practice, whether within hospitals or within physician offices. A major premise of this book is that evaluation activities should be expanded.

2
Historical Perspective on Technology in Medicine

> It has been said that though God cannot alter the past, historians can; it is perhaps because they can be useful to him in this respect that He tolerates their existence.
>
> Samuel Butler

The first goal of this chapter is to present a brief history of medical technology and its relation to the health care system. A key point to be recognized is that the medical care system developed with little technology. Most systems (for example, transportation) develop after technology is available. The medical care system was not designed to deliver cost-effective technology to patients. Instead, technology has gradually crept into practice with little or no rational planning. The result is that many technologies tend to be overused—or at least are used in circumstances that cannot be justified by available knowledge of benefits. It may be useful to consider, therefore, some historical factors that have helped create the present situation. Further, evaluation techniques could have been used to guide more rational adoption and use of medical technology, but they have been little applied. Evaluation in medicine has its own history, and its failure to gain a central place in medicine is also worth looking into.

History of Technology in Medicine

The history of medical science and medical technology may be divided into three general periods: (1) an early period of slow accumulation of medical knowledge through description and empiricism, which began with the ancient Greeks or even earlier and ended with the beginning of modern scientific thought as described by Descartes in 1637 (the main triumph of Cartesian thought was the control of infectious diseases); (2) a later period characterized by the rapid development of knowledge through modern science, primarily during the 1800s and 1900s; and (3) the modern era of extended longevity, chronic diseases, and machine-based technology. Many advances extended over periods of centuries, and the periods overlap to a degree, so this scheme is not entirely satisfactory. Nonetheless, it does give a useful overall framework for examining the subject.

Early Development of Medical Science

Science deals with the development of generalizations from a body of facts. When sufficient facts are accumulated, a hypothesis is formed that has some relation to them. Further facts can confirm or apparently confirm the hypothesis, and it then becomes doctrine (Newsholme, 1927, p. 6). Doctrine or orthodoxy has perhaps been the greatest impediment to the development of scientific medicine, and it continues to be a great problem. However, early in the history of medicine, philosophical or supernatural considerations were often more important than facts in the development of doctrine, so that medical science was held back for centuries. For example, the early view that disease was caused by the gods impeded the development of knowledge.

The Greek civilization began the rejection of supernatural causes of disease. In the fifth century B.C., Hippocrates recognized disease as part of nature, and he stressed the healing powers of nature. His doctrine refused to recognize priests and astrologers as having a legitimate concern with medicine (Newsholme, 1927, p. 12). Asklepiades, Themison, and Plato focused on disease and suggested that different patterns of symptoms corresponded to specific disease entities (Sigerist, 1970, pp. 107–112). Aristotle stressed the importance of exact observation and experimentation. Galen carried out countless dissections of animals. However, as noted above, all of these observations were hindered by existing dogmas, and it was not until the publication of Andreas Vesalius' *De Corporis Humani Fabrica Libri Septum* in 1542 that modern anatomy began (Reiser, 1978, pp. 13–16). Vesalius' great achievement was to carry out dissections of human bodies and to describe carefully what he observed, even if it was in conflict with existing dogma.

Anatomy is the foundation of modern medicine, and anatomy and physiology are inseparably bound together. Thus, as anatomy developed as a discipline, physiology (the study of normal function) became possible. The nature of the circulatory system was the question that led to the great breakthrough. The ancients had believed the heart to be to the body what the sun is to the universe. Galen developed a complex theory of circulation that dominated medicine for 1500 years. It proposed a back and forth movement of the blood, similar to that of the tides. But in 1628 William Harvey published his observations on the circulation of the blood that laid the basis for modern physiology and its relation to anatomy (Sigerist, 1970, pp. 25–31).

Perhaps the final major contribution of the early stages of scientific medicine was the classification of disease. A prominent seventeenth century proponent of scientific classification of disease was Thomas Sydenham, who believed that diseases should be classified into a finite number of definite diseases. He based his descriptions of disease on patients' descriptions of their problems and on his own clinical observations. Interestingly, he resisted the idea that anatomical study could help in the diagnosis. Nonetheless, autopsies to detect pathological changes were common by the early seventeenth century. In 1761, Morgagni published his work describing the relationships between clinical illness, findings at autopsy, and pathological changes (Sigerist, 1970, pp. 121–126).

The invention of the microscope made further understanding of the human body possible. Malpighi and Leeuwenhoek carried out early studies in the seventeenth century. In 1839, Schwann discovered that the animal organism is made up of cells (Sigerist, 1970, pp. 13–14). Virchow, building on this earlier work, developed a dynamic view of disease, emphasizing the importance of understanding physiology (Reiser, 1978, pp. 78–80). As additional specific tools for diagnosis developed in the 1700s and 1800s, classification became more and more rational, and diagnosis became more and more scientific.

Therapy was limited during the early history of medicine. Treatment with drugs is certainly one of the oldest therapeutic methods, yet less than two dozen effective drugs were known before the year 1700. About that time, for example, Robert Boyle, an early noted chemist, treated his patients with powdered cow dung for eye infection (Dowling, 1970, p. 14–16).

It was difficult to tell whether a single drug had, in fact, had an effect on a given disease, so the store of drugs grew continually with few restraints. However, the idea that specific drugs produced specific actions gradually developed and was facilitated by the introduction of new medicines, such as quinine from America in the seventeenth century (Sigerist, 1970, pp. 240–246).

Another therapy available from ancient times was surgery. The Hippocratic surgeon trephined (surgically opened) the skull, opened the abdomen and thorax, and burned hemorrhoids (Sigerist, 1970, pp. 261–266). The development of anatomy had a great effect on surgery, since the greater the knowledge of anatomy, the greater the potential of surgery. As surgery gradually became somewhat more effective, the prestige of the surgeon also began to change. He had been merely a technician or artisan, but he now became a physician. Nonetheless, until recent times, surgery was greatly hampered by two problems: the pain caused to the patient and the high rate of infection of wounds.

Beginning of Modern Scientific Medicine

The principles of modern science were laid down in 1637 by the French philosopher, Rene Descartes. His most important principles were 1) *to doubt everything that could be doubted*. He discarded speculation that had explained the behavior of the universe through final ends (e.g., the intent of a divinity) and emphasized areas where it seemed possible to develop knowledge; 2) *to separate the mind from the body*, thereby escaping medieval theology and its fatalism; and 3) *to study the biological organism as a mechanism or a machine* (Freymann, 1974, p. 51).

As this Cartesian paradigm began to be accepted, it became conceptually possible to intervene in human disasters, including disease. Thomas (1971, p. 658) notes, "The difference between the eighteenth and sixteenth centuries lies not in achievement but in aspiration." Knowledge had slowly accumulated for centuries. Yet great discoveries, such as Harvey's description of the circulation of the blood, had had little effect. "The change which occurred in the 17th century was thus not so much technological as mental. In many different spheres of life the period saw the emergence of a new faith in the potentialities of human initiative" (Thomas, 1971, p. 661).

The medical model that developed from Cartesian thought was that every disease has a single specific cause. Under this paradigm, medical science developed rapidly during the 1700s and 1800s. Auenbrugger extended the physical examination beyond superficial examination of the patient's body by striking the body with his fingers to produce sounds that gave him information about organs contained within. This technique became known as percussion (Sigerist, 1970, p. 226; Reiser, 1978, pp. 20–22). In 1816 Laennec extended the physical examination further, with his invention of the stethoscope to listen to sounds within the body (Reiser, 1978, pp. 23–44). Reiser (1978) has fully described the subsequent development of the many tools of modern medicine, including the ophthalmoscope (1850); the thermometer (early 1700s); the blood pressure cuff (1876); the electrocardiograph (1901); and the laryngoscope (1857).

The use of chemistry as a part of the diagnosis of disease also began during this period. Although, traditionally, the urine had been examined, it was the significant advances in the science of chemistry in the latter half of the 18th century that made scientific examinations possible. During the late 1700s, chemical analyses demonstrated sugar in the urine of diabetics. Tests of the blood were developed, and stomach acid was often measured by 1890 (Reiser, 1978, pp. 133–143). The microscope also had a profound effect on diagnosis, following Virchow's work. In 1843 Andral's *Pathological Hematology* described the normal components of the blood and their proportions. The term "clinical pathology" was coined in the late 1800s to describe the use of chemical, microscopical, and bacteriological techniques to study disease.

Another important diagnostic technology is the x-ray, discovered by Roentgen in 1895 and rapidly accepted by the medical profession (Reiser, 1978, pp. 58–67). The low cost of the machine and the simplicity of the process helped lead to its rapid spread. X-rays further objectified diagnosis, making it possible to look within the body. With the development of dense materials that showed white on the x-ray picture, visualizing the gastrointestinal tract became possible. By 1910, bismuth was being used to explore the human intestine from end to end. Of all the instruments of visual diagnosis, the x-ray produced the most significant changes in the methods physicians use to evaluate illness. Here was a machine directly challenging the value of touching, listening to, and talking to the patient in the diagnosis of disease. The x-ray was so widely accepted that when reports that x-rays could destroy organic life and produce damage to the skin began to appear by 1900, these harmful effects were played down by many physicians. Physicians confidently asserted that x-ray injury was unusual and was produced principally by unskilled use.

This initial great transformation in medical diagnosis engendered by the use of modern technology was not complete until the field of bacteriology developed (Reiser, 1978, pp. 82–90). Use of the microscope made possible the demonstration of microorganisms in diseased tissues. Pasteur conclusively demonstrated that spontaneous generation of microorganisms, which was the era's major doctrine to explain their presence in tissues, does not occur (Sigerist, 1970, p. 201). Koch was another important investigator who worked on a number of diseases, including anthrax and tuberculosis. He proved in the 1880s that tuberculosis was produced by a microorganism, which he named the *tubercle bacillus*. As the field developed and other investigators joined in the chase, by the beginning of the twentieth century microorganisms had been implicated as causal in a number of diseases, including pneumonia, plague, typhoid fever, diphtheria, gonorrhea, cholera, influenza, and malaria. The development of bacteriology opened the possibility of preventing disease through environmental changes and immunization, and also fostered the further development of surgery.

The sanitary revolution of the nineteenth century, a systematic intervention in the physical environment, was built on ecological approaches to disease prevention begun by the Greeks (Sigerist, 1970, pp. 289–293). Even without specific knowledge, the interventionist attitude of the nineteenth century led to great reforms. Whole towns were torn down and rebuilt, new water and drainage systems developed, and the purity of food was controlled (Rosen, 1976). The scientific knowledge gained by Pasteur and others made hygiene even more effective.

Perhaps the greatest advance, however, and the one leading to this period's being called the "Age of Pasteur," was specific immunization against disease. The idea of immunity to infection is an old one (Sigerist, 1970, pp. 285–288). It has long been known that a person who had one attack of smallpox would not have another. This knowledge led to attempts to infect healthy people purposely during a light epidemic of a disease. In India, children were wrapped in clothes that had been worn by those with smallpox. Jenner believed that infection with the benign cowpox protected against smallpox. He tested this theory in 1796 by vaccinating a boy with cowpox organisms. The boy's resultant immunity to smallpox was then demonstrated.

Pasteur's contributions were equally dramatic (Sigerist, 1970, pp. 285–288). He weakened organisms to develop vaccines for chicken cholera, anthrax, and swine fever, and then for rabies. The techniques developed by Pasteur made possible immunization against such common diseases as diphtheria and tetanus. The isolation of viruses in 1935 and their subsequent growth in cell culture made possible the development of vaccines for poliomyelitis, measles, rubella (German measles), and influenza.

The development of surgery was also accelerated as a result of bacteriology. Semmelweiss had concluded that postpartum fever was a wound infection disease and had required all examining physicians to disinfect their hands in chlorine water before examining patients on his obstetrics wards (Sigerist, 1970, pp. 201–204). Lister demonstrated that he could prevent infection by applying chemical disinfectants to the surgical wound and its dressing. Physical disinfection gradually took over, and only objects that had been boiled in water or sterilized by steam were allowed to come into contact with the wound. With the discovery by Davy that the gas nitrous oxide was an effective narcotic, and the demonstration by Wells in 1844 that the gas made extraction of a tooth painless, surgery became a more acceptable intervention (Sigerist, 1970, pp. 266–268). The development of modern surgery had begun.

The development of chemistry stimulated the beginnings of modern pharmacology. Organic chemical substances such as morphine were isolated from plants. It was now becoming clear that specific chemicals had specific effects (Sigerist, 1970, p. 248). As a result, dosages, side effects, and effects on disease were studied. In 1860, salicylic acid was synthesized from coal tar. By the end of the nineteenth century, the extraction of the active elements of drugs and synthesis of new chemical substances were established as the basis for modern pharmacology (Dowling, 1970, pp. 16–17). An early dramatic application of the new principles was the development, by Ehrlich in 1911, of Salvarsan for the treatment of syphilis. This was the so-called "magic bullet" (Sigerist, 1970, pp. 248–249). Discovery that a red dye, Prontosil rubrum, protected animals from streptococcal disease led to the introduction of sulfa drugs in 1936. Not only were the sulfa drugs of importance themselves, but they inspired further research. Penicillin was introduced in 1943, followed by streptomycin. For the first time, it was possible to treat effectively such infectious diseases as pneumonia, middle ear infection, and strep throat, which may lead to rheumatic fever. Mahoney (1959, p. 14) quotes Sir Henry Dale on the implications of these advances: "Look back, those who can do so, to the beginning of this century and recall again the state of medicinal treatment fifty years ago. . . . The idea that a remedy could directly remove or neutralize the cause of an illness was still a startling innovation, and neither physician nor patient had yet learned to expect a medication which would go thus to the root of the trouble. . . . This aspect of medicine, at least, has been the subject of a greater advance since this century began than in all the centuries which went before it. . . ."

If the developments described above or that follow below seem logical, linear, and organized, that is the danger of a brief historical sketch. A more complete and lengthy telling of the story could bring out the dead ends, the resistance to new ideas, the advances made by chance, the possibilities lost through poor communication, and so on. Chapter 3 will shed some additional light on the process of medical advance.

Modern Developments

Chapter 1 mentioned that, as infectious diseases have been controlled, chronic diseases have come to prominence. Because they are more complex in their etiology, their control has not been nearly so successful. Halfway technology has been the result.

Since 1950 there has been an explosion of biomedical knowledge. The discovery of the structure of DNA set off a biological revolution. Medicine has been transformed; entirely new disciplines and specialties have been developed (President's Biomedical Research Panel, 1976; Handler, 1970). However, as mentioned earlier, the value of this scientific information for the health of the population is far from clear.

Whatever its effect, the technology of medicine has changed rather dramatically. For example, fewer than one hundred types of chemical laboratory tests were performed 25 years ago, while at least 600 different examinations are performed now (Brownfield and Ives, 1976). New imaging devices such as the computed tomography (CT) scanner have radically changed the process of diagnosis. New operative technology has made open-heart surgery relatively safe. Prosthetic devices and organ transplants are common. Monitoring of a variety of physiological functions is done more and more frequently on hospitalized patients, especially those admitted to an ever-growing number of specialized intensive care units. Even monitoring at home is becoming fairly common. Hospitals have changed correspondingly to incorporate this technology.

Historical Roots of Technology-Dependent Medical Care

The preceding history is primarily descriptive. The medical developments described, however, cannot be considered in static isolation. The processes and the results of the historical development of modern medical technology, influenced by and combining with other historical factors of our society, are important determinants of the current situation in medicine and its technology. This section will examine some of those more dynamic relationships. Chapter 8 expands upon this section through its discussion of current factors influencing the use of medical technology.

Cartesian Thought

As discussed in the preceding section, Cartesian thought was a major impetus to the development of modern scientific medicine. But Cartesian thought has had significant, and increasingly important, negative consequences. The Cartesian paradigm of one cause for one disease does not apply well to chronic diseases and their complex etiology. Nor is the separation of body and mind a helpful paradigm in the modern age. As Freymann (1974, p. 9) said, "The Cartesian physician tended to forget that not everything we can count counts, nor can everything that counts be counted." The mechanistic Cartesian view has led to much wasted effort and money and has fostered a system skewed to hospital-based, technology-dependent medical care. Cartesian thought leads one to concentrate on what is tangible and to ignore the more complex variables that cannot be quantified, such as social and behavioral factors. It fosters an engineering approach to medicine that in turn leads to coronary care units rather than programs to prevent heart disease.

Medicine as a Profession

The concept of a physician influenced and was influenced by many historical factors, among them the emergence of medical technology. In early years, physicians had few effective tools, often received very little pay, and frequently engaged in medicine as a part-time occupation. Their reputation, income, and sense of profession have increased along with the development of technologies. It is difficult to say which are the causal factors and which the result. Most likely, subtle intersections of these factors with other social factors (such as insurance) changed these factors in some reinforcing, interactive way. One thing, however, is clear: The concept of medicine as a profession is heavily dependent on physicians as the wielders of a complex arsenal of technology.

The tremendous growth in knowledge in the nineteenth century led to specialization of physicians, both in research and practice. As in the case of surgeons, specialization brought higher prestige and higher incomes. By the 1880s, specialties were growing rapidly, and by 1929, almost one out of four private practitioners in the United States was a full-time specialist. Other factors accelerated the move to specialization: Urbanization led to concentrations of people that could support specialists; physicians desired more regular hours and better pay; and there were no legal, social, or professional barriers to prevent specialists from competing with generalists for patients. Finally, the developing technology of medicine, such as x-rays, in itself stimulated the development of new specialties.

Medical Education

In ancient Greece, physicians learned their profession by apprenticeship (Sigerist, 1970, p. 300). Much of this tradition survives in medical education. The physician-in-training, while under supervision of more senior physicians, observes many individual patients with a given disease condition. Medical diagnosis and treatment are so complex that much cannot be encompassed in textbooks. The physician faced with a patient problem tends to think in terms of his or her experience.

The emphasis on apprenticeship, however, began to diminish somewhat as the universities began to develop in the Middle Ages and medical instruction became more formal (Sigerist, 1970, pp. 301–304).

In the early history of the United States, medical education was still largely imparted by apprenticeship. However, in the decades after the Flexner Report on medical education in 1910, medical education in the United States changed to the basic form it has today: hospital-based, with a heavy emphasis on biomedical science and technology presented by a full-time medical faculty who are themselves biomedical researchers and medical specialists (Banta, 1971; Ebert, 1977). At the same time, as Jonas shows, the scientific method is not taught (Jonas, 1978, pp. 211, 213). The student is not taught the first of Descartes' tenets: to doubt everything that can be doubted. Instead, the medical student is taught by specialists who depend on medical technology for their livelihood.

Organization of Medical Care

The technology of medicine has also interacted with the structure of medical care. Structure or organization of health care affects the use of medical technologies; likewise the historical development of technology has affected organization of practice and institutions.

In the Middle Ages, the physician practiced alone and rarely had a connection with a hospital. With the growth in scientific knowledge in the sixteenth and seventeenth centuries, physicians were increasingly brought into hospitals as salaried members. In European countries, the development of social insurance (see next section) facilitated transition to a health service covering the entire population on a compulsory basis, and nationalization of private hospitals to maximize planning and coordination. The new knowledge of the cause of infectious diseases and a lessening of the fear of infection in hospitals combined to encourage the use of hospitals, and these institutions became the home of the rapidly developing technology of medical care (Knowles, 1973). In part, the expense of the new technology forced such an institutional base. By the early 1900s, these changes brought the middle and upper classes into what previously had been an institution for the poor (Rosen, 1963).

Similar forces have been factors in the increase in group practices and the growing percentage of physicians on salary in the United States. Although many physicians have resisted these changes, the need for access to x-ray and laboratory tests and for consultation with specialists has stimulated physicians to become part of larger institutions. The search, informal as it is, to discover the best system of practice to satisfy these technology-based needs and still accommodate other factors (such as close relationships with patients, or flexibility in practice management) still goes on.

Financing of Medical Care

In early society the physician was paid according to the success of the treatment (Sigerist, 1970, pp. 308–310). Fees continued to be common during the Middle Ages, but other modes of payment developed as well. "Sick funds" developed as insurance to spread the risks of illness and prepay the costs of care. These private associations either formed for medical care purposes, or, in the case of guilds or religious societies, existed for other reasons as well. The poor generally did without physician services.

In the last half of the nineteenth century, a fundamental change occurred in financing with the development of social insurance (Abel-Smith, 1964). Industrialization, with better education and relative prosperity, along with the growing credibility of medical care, led to expanded financial coverage for service. Through worker pressure, social insurance was inaugurated in Germany in 1881, and the model developed there was followed by practically all other European governments. The result was a marked increase in the number of physicians and hospitals.

In the United States, the development of the employer-employee benefit funds since World War II is somewhat analogous to the development of social insurance in Europe (Banta and Bosch, 1974). With Medicare coverage for the elderly, Medicaid coverage for the poor, and employment-related coverage for workers and their families, the technology of medicine is available to the vast majority of U.S. citizens.

Technology as Commodity: Emergence of the Drug and Device Industry

The development of pharmacology in the 1800s and the increasing possibilities of synthesizing drugs led to the development of industry involvement. The Civil War provided an impetus because of the associated sharp growth in demand for drugs. E. R. Squibb & Sons; Sharp and Dohme; Parke, Davis & Company; and Eli Lilly and Company were all founded at about that time. Insulin and the development of vitamins gave the industry new products in the 1900s (Mahoney, 1959, p. 10). World War II stimulated further development of the industry, as it made the transition from bulk supplier to supplier of pills and capsules. The development of penicillin and the broad-spectrum antibiotics in the postwar period ended the domination of the market by established firms, and the potential for profits encouraged a number of new companies to enter the pharmaceutical field. Between 1951 and 1960, more than 3800 new products and dosage forms were introduced into the U.S. market. It has been estimated that 90 percent of the prescriptions written in 1965 were for drugs unknown in 1950 (Schnee and Caglarcan, 1978).

There are now about 800 U.S. drug companies that produce and sell drugs for the prescription drug market. Growth of the industry is shown by the increase in annual sales for the United States alone from about $1 billion in 1950 to almost $9 billion in 1976 (Silverman and Lee, 1974, pp. 26–27; Schnee and Caglarcan, 1978). Worldwide sales of U.S. prescription drugs have risen rapidly as well, reaching about $3 billion in 1972.

The industry that produces medical devices and products has also developed since World War II. The war stimulated development of new devices that subsequently found application in the medical area. Ultrasound is one example.

Also of great importance was the fostering of the field of bioengineering. In the immediate postwar period, a number of devices were invented that revolutionized medical care and had significant implications for costs. In 1951, Leonard Skeggs built a prototype automated blood chemistry analyzer, subsequently marketed by Technicon Corporation as the Sequential Multiple-Analyzer (SMA). In 1969, Technicon sold 18,000 analyzers, and by 1972 more than 50 percent of hospitals had automated their chemistry laboratories (OTA, 1976, pp. 10–11). Another innovation that subsequently had profound implications was renal dialysis. Willem Kolff built the first machine in the early 1930s. The invention of the "Schribner shunt" in 1960 made long-term dialysis possible. The 1972 Social Security Amendments extended coverage to all those with end-stage renal disease, and the costs to the nation are approaching $1 billion a year (OTA, 1976, pp. 17–18). The advances during World War II in instrumentation and electronics as well as surgery made long-term cardiac pacemakers possible. In the United States, the first totally implantable pacemaker was placed in a patient with heart block in 1960. Medtronics introduced the device shortly thereafter, and other companies followed. About 75,000 units were sold in the United States during 1975, and worldwide sales were estimated to be 147,000 units, with a gross business of $200 million a year (OTA, 1976, pp. 19–20). The result of such advances and of the large market for devices is that there are now more than 2,000 manufacturers of medical devices.

Thus, the drug and device revolutions have occurred largely since 1945, and the sizeable profits and political power of the companies have increased correspondingly (Waitzkin, 1979).

Government Support for Biomedical Research

Substantial Federal government support for biomedical research and medical technology development also effectively began with World War II. A

Federal Committee on Medical Research established by President Roosevelt coordinated a research effort whose results were impressive (Strickland, 1972, p. 15–16). In the postwar period, the National Institutes of Health was formed, and new institutes were added to it almost yearly. During the 1950s, NIH's growth was phenomenal, so much so that by 1965 NIH made up more than 37 percent of the entire Federal health budget (House of Representatives, 1976a, pp. 14–16). This percentage has dropped because of the tremendous growth of Medicare and Medicaid, but the absolute *amount* of support has continued to rise. The fruits of the research supported the medical technological revolution.

Not only did the support for biomedical research in itself foster development, but it supported medical schools. From 1948 to 1958, the number of medical school faculty members doubled (Jonas, 1978, p. 245). The result was a medical education process focusing on research and specialized medical care, as described in a previous section.

Historical View of the Evaluation of Medical Technology

Throughout recorded history, physicians have made observations on the effects of new treatments on patients. As Hill (1962) notes, "Even the witch-doctor trying out for the first time a new and nauseating compound must surely, like Alice nibbling at the mushroom in Wonderland, have murmured to himself 'which way?' . . . Such personal observations of a handful of patients, acutely made and accurately recorded by the masters of clinical medicine, have been, and will continue to be, fundamental to the progress of medicine."

Credit for carrying out the first controlled clinical trial goes to John Lind, who tested a number of "cures" for scurvy in 1747. Although Lind's trial was small, it yielded powerful evidence for the efficacy of orange and lemon juices. It is interesting to note that the results of this trial were not used to affect policy towards the diet of seamen until 40 years later (Lambert, 1978, pp. 139–140). Another careful trial was that of Pierre Louis in Paris in 1835. Louis studied the effects of bloodletting on pneumonia, erysipelas, and inflammation of the throat, and found no differences in mortality or in duration of disease between patients bled and patients not bled. This study was very controversial at the time, but eventually it did help lead to abandonment of the practice of bloodletting. It is also worth noting that Louis believed in bloodletting and was dubious about his results (Lambert, 1978, p. 141).

Statistics and probability techniques were available as early as the eighteeenth century. In 1721, for example, Cotton Mather reported that, in the Boston smallpox epidemic of that year, more than 1 in 6 people who were not inoculated against the disease died, but that only about 1 in 60 who were inoculated did so (Shryock, 1969).

Although quantitative evaluation of medical technology demonstrated in the late 1800s that many interventions were not effective and led to the decline of accepted treatments and (temporarily) of the confidence of the public in medicine, the "Age of Pasteur" brought a revolution in medical technology. During the early part of the 1900s, scientific evaluation of efficacy and safety was not regarded as a critical aspect of medicine. The main reasons, probably, were the successes of Pasteur and others and the high level of public confidence in physicians.

Nonetheless, techniques continually improved, and Hill was able to formulate the principles and requirements for a well-designed controlled clinical trial in 1937 (Hill, 1937).

It was in part the availability of these research methods that led the Congress to react to the sulfanilamide disaster[1] of the late 1930s with a law requiring the demonstration of the safety of drugs before they could be marketed in the United States (Lambert, 1978, pp. 158–160). The 1962 amendments to this law added the requirement that efficacy be demonstrated, and in 1976, regulation of the safety and efficacy of medical devices was also required.

Why has evaluation not been an integral part of medical technology development and use? Lambert suggested that there have been three main reasons historically: (1) reverence for authority and tradition; (2) lack of effective remedies; and (3) the relationship of doctor and patient. We now have many effective remedies. Therefore, in a reversal of the second factor, past dramatic successes seem a modern reason for the lack of demand for evaluations. The most important force, though, is probably the power of doctrine, of the existing paradigm. By and large, physicians do not doubt.

---

[1]Sulfanilamide, a synthetic chemical demonstrated to be of great value in treating such conditions as streptococcal septicemia, came into general use in the U.S. in 1937. This chemical and its family of sulfonamides were hailed as miracle drugs. In that year a small drug company marketed an "Elixir of Sulfanilimide." Hundreds of gallons were distributed. Physicians began noticing that many patients taking the compound suffered kidney failure. A rapid and joint effort by the public and private health sectors established that the patients had severe toxic liver damage, identified the poisonous element of the compound, and stopped subsequent distribution and use of the Elixir. The poison was diethylene glycol, and it was the solvent used to carry the sulfanilamide in the Elixir. The hard data: "Altogether, 358 persons were poisoned . . . 107 died, many of them children. The chemist involved committed suicide" (Lambert, 1978, pp. 53–55).

They need to believe that the services that they provide are of benefit, just as patients need to believe that they are benefited.[2] This psychological need limits the value of clinical experience and requires good controlled studies. It also causes physicians to resist withholding even unproved treatments from control groups. As Lambert said, "The admission of doubt and ignorance is essential in order to recognize the need for controlled trials" (1978, pp. 143–144).

Connections

This chapter has presented three interwoven histories: (1) that of the development of technology in medicine; (2) that of other aspects of medical care and society; and (3) that of evaluation. The present role of technology in health care arises from all these historical and cultural roots. Although it would take volumes of space and knowledge beyond ours to adequately discuss the integration of the three histories, we feel it is important to present the flavor of that integration:

With the development of knowledge in the 1800s, infectious disease was largely controlled. The development of the "miracle drugs" of the 1940s and 1950s further encouraged the hope that there would be a technological solution to every medical problem. Industry moved into the developing market and found ready acceptance among physicians not trained to evaluate technology. The combined political pressure of providers, consumers, and industry has led to third-party insurance coverage (without the coordinated planning systems that developed in Europe) of much of U.S. medical care. In short, historical developments have all encouraged the rapid diffusion of medical technology without careful consideration of its benefits, risks, and costs. Because of the faith in technology, as well as other factors, available evaluative techniques have not been used aggressively.

In summary, the technology of the medical care system includes a class of older technologies that were not evaluated as they entered the system because there was nothing else to offer the patient, and a class of newer technologies that have entered the system because of the faith engendered by earlier technological successes. Because neither class of medical technology has been adequately evaluated, we are left knowing little about their value.

[2]On the other hand, it should be noted that these factors are also in large part responsible for the placebo effect, a strong and often successful aspect of the practice of medicine.

3
Research and Development

> Next to nature there is nothing more wonderful than man's gradual understanding of it.
>
> George Sarton

This chapter depicts research and development as a two-stage process: basic research, and applied research and development. It discusses some of the difficulties in defining basic research and in clearly differentiating between basic and applied research projects. It presents an overview of societal support of health research and development. Finally, it describes some proposed changes in processes for supporting such research.

The Process of Research and Development

Basic Research

Medical advance rests on an expanding foundation of knowledge about the biological mechanisms that underlie the normal functioning of the human body and its malfunction in disease. This knowledge is acquired largely through basic biological research (American Biology Council, 1972).

Lacking sophisticated tools, general theories, and the framework of the scientific method, early biologists (as described in Chapter 2) were restricted to careful observation and extensive classification. Occasionally, general explanatory theories (for example, Darwin's theory of evolution or Harvey's theory of the circulation) emerged from the compilation of numerous observations. Most often, though, the early biologists amassed bodies of information that awaited further progress for their interpretation.

In the twentieth century, biology has matured as an experimental science. Earlier detailed and reliable descriptions of whole animals or organs provided frameworks that have allowed the formulation and testing of hypotheses about the mechanisms that underlie a variety of phenomena previously described but not understood. The availability of new ideas and tools, derived largely from advances in the physical sciences, made it possible for biologists to gain insight into many organic processes by focusing on smaller and smaller parts of the whole animal. Refinements in the techniques of microscopy and the later advent of electron microscopy allowed examination not only of the cells from which tissues are built but also of subcellular elements. Applications of chemical theories and techniques to biological problems has made possible the study of the molecules and reactions from which all biological structures and functions are derived. The resulting progress, sometimes through spectacular breakthroughs, but more often as a result of plodding, methodical work, has led to an understanding of the mechanisms that underlie a number of important and intuitively fascinating biological phenomena. Among the triumphs of modern biology are the discoveries of:

The molecules and reactions responsible for the transmission of inherited characteristics from one generation to the next;

The way in which chemical energy is transformed to mechanical energy to permit muscular contractions; and

The ways in which large molecules called enzymes act as catalysts to regulate the chemical reactions of the body.

The promise of such basic research is eventual advance in the prevention, diagnosis, and treatment of diseases. Two related assumptions underlie arguments in defense of basic research. First, biologists assume that knowledge acquired from studies of lower animals (which are readily available, provide numerous technically advantageous features, and can ethically be subjected to experimentation) will be applicable to humans. Second, they assume that knowledge about the normal functioning of the human body will lead to an understanding of the body's malfunction in disease. As biological knowledge has accumulated, these assumptions have been generally confirmed. Knowledge acquired through basic biological research has led to the development of effective and beneficial medical technologies. In some cases, such understanding has allowed the development of technologies such as vaccines, which prevent disease and make expensive, risky, and only partially effective treatment unnecessary.

The application of basic research findings can occur in several ways. Frequently, the immediate connection between basic research and its eventual applications is not clear, as when medical benefit is derived from the confluence of seemingly unrelated lines of research.

Research on anatomy and physiology when combined with the invention of the microscope (which was done out of curiosity) made modern medicine possible.

In many other cases, logical progression from basic research to its applications can be discerned retrospectively, although such applications might not have been predictable in advance.

Biochemical studies on metabolism led to the discovery of enzymes that regulate metabolic processes, then to studies of enzyme deficiencies in disease states, and finally to the use of enzyme assays as important diagnostic tools.

Occasionally, medical advance comes serendipitously from lines of biological research far removed from the particular medical area that benefits.

The discovery of the Rh factor in blood, which led eventually to prevention of the fatal syndrome, erythroblastosis fetalis, resulted from work on variations in the color of butterfly wings (Comroe and Dripps, 1974).

The technique of freeze drying, now widely used to preserve antibiotics and blood fractions without loss of potency, was developed in studies on the water content of liver and muscle (Comroe and Dripps, 1974).

Basic research in physics and chemistry also can lead to medical advances. Sometimes the application of research findings in the physical sciences is rapid, as when Roentgen discovered x-rays while studying the electrical nature of matter and quickly applied his discovery to the examination of human tissue (Comroe and Dripps, 1974). More often, however, the physical sciences supply background, theories, techniques, and tools that subsequently are used for conducting biological research or for applying biological knowledge to practical ends.

Applied Research and Development

In its Forward Plan for Health, HHS (then HEW) defined "applied research and development" in biomedicine as "activity drawing upon basic information to create solutions to problems in prevention, treatment, or cure of disease" (Public Health Service, 1975). While basic research in biology seeks to understand vital processes, applied research seeks their manipulation or control.

An illustration of the difference between basic and applied research is provided by the recent work of Bruce Ames and his collaborators at the University of California at Berkeley (McCann and Ames, 1976). For a number of years, Ames was engaged in studies on molecular biology. He created and used mutant strains of bacteria to study the mechanisms of genetic control of metabolic processes. This work was, by definition, basic research. At some point, Ames realized that the information he and others had gathered about genetic mechanisms, and the bacterial mutants he had created, could be used to determine whether particular chemicals were mutagenic—i.e., whether they caused mutations. This information, he realized, would be valuable because other researchers had found that most carcinogenic chemicals are also mutagenic. (In fact, chemicals may cause cancer by inducing mutations.) He therefore developed such an assay and has since used it to screen a wide variety of industrial and environmental compounds for potential carcinogenicity. Ames' application of knowledge gained through his earlier work to the practical end of developing a test for carcinogens is an example of applied research.

The vitality of applied research varies from field to field, as a function of the extent and strength of the knowledge base. Knowledge acquired through biochemical and physiological research has been applied to the development of many medical technologies. Ames' work on the application of molecular biology to practical ends is particularly noteworthy because the field of molecular biology is so new—the discipline has existed for only a few decades.

Although further application of recently acquired knowledge can be anticipated, it is a mistake to:

> attribute to biology and medicine a much greater store of usable information than actually exists. In real life, the biomedical sciences have not yet reached the stage of general applicability to disease mechanisms. In some respects we are like the physical sciences of the early twentieth century, booming along into new territory, but without an equivalent for the engineering of that time. It is possible that we are on the verge of developing a proper applied science, but it has to be said we don't have one yet [Thomas, 1974, p. 116]

Much of the applied research that contributes to the development of medical technologies is not, strictly speaking, biological. Rather, it results from the application of knowledge derived from the physical sciences to the solution of biological problems. For example, chemical engineers are engaged in developing "biomaterials" that neither damage nor are damaged by the environment of the human body and thus can be used in invasive medical procedures or for implants. The technology of electronics has provided many tools. For example, instruments for measuring biological parameters have been adapted for diagnostic uses, such as the continuous-flow blood analyzer and the CT scanner. Also, miniaturized power sources and control elements are being used in therapeutic devices such as the cardiac pacemaker and prototypes of the implantable artificial heart. Microcomputers are beginning to find a wide variety of medical applications. Organic chemists have developed techniques and strategies for synthesizing compounds that might be used as drugs.

Although applied research of these types is, by definition, goal-oriented, the development of a specific new medical technology is not always the immediate goal. Applied researchers in both biological and physical sciences frequently concentrate on the development of new materials, tools, or techniques that they assume will be useful for a variety of applications.

The targeted development of a new technology begins when knowledge derived from basic and applied research is sufficient to support the effort. Although such development is not without risks, both human and financial, the eventual outcome can be predicted with some assurance, if a solid foundation has been established by prior research. As Thomas (1974, p. 118) argues,

> When you are organized to apply knowledge, set up targets, produce a usable product, you require . . . certainty from the outset. All the facts on which you base protocols must be reasonably hard facts, with unambiguous meaning. The challenge is to plan the work and organize the workers so that it will come out precisely as predicted. . . . You need the intelligible basic facts to begin with.

It must be emphasized, though, that there are many sources of these facts. Workers engaged in developing new technologies, whether they be biologists, engineers, or physicians, draw on knowledge gained through basic and applied research in biological and physical sciences alike, as well as on the rich lore of industrial, experimental, epidemiological, and clinical experience.

Complexities in the Process of Technology Development

The categories distinguished above—basic research, and applied research and development—are adequate to classify a large number of the activities that precede widespread acceptance of a new medical technology. Categories similar to those presented here are commonly used in making decisions about resource allocation for biomedical R&D, establishing policies and priorities, and organizing institutional capabilities. However, such a classification scheme is highly idealized. At least two severe limitations to the scheme must be considered.

First, the history of science and medicine shows that basic research, applied research, development, and even diffusion often progress simultaneously and not sequentially (Carter et al., 1976). Investigators approach the development of new technologies from many viewpoints and often independently; useful innovation most often results from the confluence of separate streams of basic, applied, and clinical research. Also, later steps in the process feed back on earlier ones—for example, new technologies may make new types of research possible, or clinical experience may suggest fruitful new research possibilities. Retrospective studies may discover—or even impose—a logical order that could not have been discerned while development was in progress. Thus, programs of assessment may aim for, but not always achieve, examination of the development of new medical technologies "at the earliest possible point."

Second, many R&D programs cannot readily be fitted into one of the categories: basic research or applied research and development. The boundaries between categories are fluid, creating problems in understanding the R&D process and in attempting assessment or control. Although one can do little to sharpen these boundaries, one can point out why and in what ways they are indistinct.

Basic Versus Applied Research

Many types of research can easily be classified as basic research, and others, as applied. There is a vast middle ground, however, that cannot be easily classified.

One problem in defining basic and applied research on biological systems can be illustrated by comparing biology with the physical sciences. Physics and chemistry are both sufficiently mature to support "theoretical" enterprises, which deal entirely with abstractions, usually mathematically. Biological processes, in contrast, have not yet been adequately described and cataloged, a prerequisite to the creation of a firm, predictive theoretical base. This is not to say that biological principles of great generality have not been discovered—they have. With few exceptions, however, biologists are still experimentalists; they are not theoreticians.

Biology and the physical sciences differ at the other end of the R&D spectrum as well. Often, massive pieces of capital equipment are developed by engineers from a base of knowledge in chemistry and physics. Prototypes must be built in industrial laboratories and often require organization and resources on an industrial scale. Medical technologies are, however, usually small enough to be built with limited resources in the laboratory or at the medical center by small groups of workers; pilot plants are seldom required. Development of medical technologies may of course be enormously expensive, but the physical scale is limited.

Thus, many research activities in the physical sciences are theoretical and, therefore, indisputably basic, or are industrial in orientation and scale and therefore clearly applied. In biology, most research activities fall into a middle ground where classification is more difficult.

There are other problems of classification as well. Basic research is usually defined as an attempt to understand nature, while applied research is seen as an attempt to control nature. However, the aims of a particular project and its outcomes may be significantly different. Basic researchers sometimes acquire knowledge or devise techniques that have immediate applicability; applied researchers frequently make discoveries that lead to new understanding. Furthermore, the very concept of experimental science runs contrary to the distinction between understanding and control. Basic researchers must devise ways to manipulate nature if they are to perform experiments. The techniques they develop may have immediate practical as well as experimental utility.

Several attempts have been made to formulate characteristics that can adequately distinguish between basic and applied research. Lewis Thomas, for example, has claimed that "surprise is what makes the difference." He contends that basic research requires "a high degree of uncertainty; otherwise it isn't likely to be an important problem." Applied research, he feels, requires "a high degree of certainty from the outset" (1974, p. 118). Although appealing, this distinction may not be useful. It does not completely describe either the basic researcher, who is not working in a vacuum and may be quite certain of what he hopes to achieve, or the applied researcher, whose activities are also creative, intellectually challenging and, in fact, sometimes quite uncertain.

Comroe and Dripps, in a study of the sources of knowledge that lead to medical innovation, make the distinction between "clinically oriented" and "non-clinically oriented" research (1974, 1976). However, since funding agencies stress clinical relevance in their application forms, and since all biological research is potentially relevant, the purported orientation of a research project or publication does not seem to be useful in devising a meaningful distinction. A study by the Batelle Columbus Laboratories, with aims similar to the work of Comroe and Dripps, distinguishes between "mission-oriented" and "nonmission-oriented" research. This distinction, which is sometimes used by the NIH in describing its programs, is subject to the same caveats as is that of Comroe and Dripps.

Thus, although some research programs can easily be classified as "basic" or "applied," there are many activities that defy categorization. This fuzzy line creates great problems for those contemplating technology evaluations. On one hand, "basic" research can masquerade as "applied" research to compete for funding in an increasingly goal-oriented system; on the other hand, "applied" research can masquerade as "basic" research to escape the pressures of social accountability that increase as one gets closer to practical application of knowledge.

Applied Research and Clinical Testing

Applied research performed in vitro (outside of the body) or with animals raises fundamentally different problems from those raised in clinical testing on humans, and different forms of assessment are appropriate for these two types of activities. Ideally, applied research and development of new medical technologies would depend largely on animal tests, with clinical testing on humans occurring only when development is thought to be complete. However, testing on humans is sometimes required well before a new technology has been completely developed. In some cases, work on animals cannot anticipate the special problems that human anatomy and physiology pose. In other cases, the uniquely human ability to respond verbally is required to assess the success of a new technology and to determine the proper directions for future developmental effort. Finally, some technologies, especially procedures, are developed by practitioners who have patients available to them, but do not have the facilities or the expertise for work on animals. For these reasons, activities of applied research and clinical testing are often inextricably linked.

Research Not Fitting Into the Classification

A major problem with the above model is that it gives a great deal of credit to the biomedical researcher and clinical physician and none to the social scientist, the statistician, or the nutritionist. Many other health workers and many other types of research have contributed to biomedical knowledge. In particular, the social sciences, nutritional research, and epidemiological research have made major contributions to the understanding of health and disease. These "non-traditional" forms of research have been underfunded and underemphasized, but are now gaining more attention

(House of Representatives, 1976a; OTA, 1979b). Further, research on chronic diseases often depends on a symbiosis between different types of research, with, for example, new laboratory methods making more important epidemiological research possible. As will be discussed in Chapter 6, epidemiological methods have been used in testing efficacy and safety of medical technologies. In addition, they have led to advances in the prevention and control of disease. The causes of such diseases as cholera, scurvy, and lung cancer have been identified through epidemiological research. For example, epidemiological data have shown that cigarette smoking is the major cause of lung cancer, so that lung cancer is almost totally preventable. Yet basic research has not discovered the mechanism by which cigarette smoking causes cancer (Breslow, 1976).

Development of Different Types of Medical Technology

Different types of medical technology are developed in different places and in different ways. These variations pose problems and must be considered if evaluation programs are to be realistic and effective. The following paragraphs describe some features unique to the development of the three categories of medical technology that were distinguished in Chapter 1: drugs, devices, and procedures.

Drugs

The link between basic biomedical research and drug development is often clear. Drugs develop from a basic knowledge of organic chemistry, pharmacology, and human pathophysiology. Occasionally, knowledge is sufficient to permit the rational design of new drugs. For example, the development of polio vaccines, which are considered drugs for purposes of this book, was based on a solid foundation of knowledge derived from basic research. Basic research in biochemistry and bacteriology has also permitted prediction of successful strategies for synthesizing some antibiotics. In many other cases, basic research has led to the development of new drugs even without complete knowledge of their mechanisms of action.

Some drug companies maintain institutes for, and support work in, biochemistry and pharmacology. However, much of the basic research that precedes the development of new drugs is supported by Federal agencies, especially NIH, and takes place in universities and medical centers. A study of 68 pharmaceutical innovations showed that over half were made possible by discoveries made outside of the drug industry—in universities, hospitals, and research institutes (Mansfield et al., 1971, p. 185). Although some applied research targeted to the development of new drugs is funded by NIH, most is supported by private industry.

Devices

Research in biomedical sciences such as physiology and anatomy provides knowledge that permits development of devices for diagnostic, preventive, and therapeutic purposes. However, much of the basic research that leads eventually to the development of devices is performed outside the biomedical research sector in such fields as physics, chemistry, and electronics. This helps to make the development and marketing of devices especially complex, and little literature is available on this process.

The successful development of devices requires a combination of expertise in both the biological and the physical sciences (Brown and Dickson, 1969). The application of the tools of mathematics and the physical sciences to biological and medical problems is called biomedical engineering (Oakes, 1975). Biomedical engineers have achieved some spectacular successes in recent years, but numerous difficulties beset their work. One is that most physicians are not trained to collaborate effectively with engineers to solve problems, or even to recognize the possibility of a technological solution. Few individuals have sufficient training in both biology (or medicine) and engineering to work alone. Also, in a marketplace oriented to profits, medical device manufacturers may develop and overproduce equipment of questionable utility or fail to support the development of types of equipment that are needed (Utterback, 1976). Additionally, engineers are trained to think in terms of physical performance characteristics and technical precision but often fail to evaluate the effect of new technologies on the health of populations or individuals. Finally, many feel that Federal health agencies are reluctant to fund private companies to conduct research or to develop new medical technologies that might return profits to those companies.

In the area of medical equipment, funding for applied research and development is largely private. There are some Federal programs to facilitate research and development of certain devices (Madjid, 1975). These are often fragmented, however, as shown by the complex pattern of Federal investment in the development of medical diagnostic ultrasound (Table 3–1). Furthermore, it is frequently difficult to document these diverse sources of funds.

Table 3-1.
Funding for Research and Development in Ultrasonic Imaging Diagnostic Instrumentation, By Federal Agency, 1975

National Bureau of Standards	$100,000
Department of Defense	
Army	120,000
Navy	285,535
Energy Research and Development Administration	80,000
Department of Health, Education, and Welfare	
Food and Drug Administration	841,459
Health Resources Administration	25,000
National Institutes of Health	
National Cancer Institute	418,514
National Heart and Lung Institute	2,851,165
National Institute of General Medical Sciences	1,530,166
National Institute of Arthritis, Metabolic and Digestive Diseases	118,964
National Eye Institute	439,297
National Institute of Neurologic and Communicative Disorders and Stroke	379,905
Division of Research Resources	20,000
Division of Research Services	50,000
Social and Rehabilitation Service	24,851
National Aeronautics and Space Administration	360,000
National Science Foundation	818,850
Veterans Administration	20,500
TOTAL	$8,484,206

Procedures

Because a procedure is a combination of technique with drugs or device, or both, its development is complex and depends on research and development in several different fields. The many bodies of knowledge and lines of research that led to the development of one complex procedure, cardiac pacemaker implantation, are shown in Figure 1-1.

Techniques themselves develop largely from knowledge gained through clinical experience; thus, advances in technique depend on creative clinicians and probably encompass thousands of small incremental changes in medical practice, which diffuse in unstudied ways.

Funding and Priority Setting for Research and Development

The major policy tool for impacting on biomedical research—and indirectly on medical technology—is funding of R & D.

Expenditures on biomedical research and the development of medical technology represent about 3.5 percent of the expenditures in the health area in the United States, or an estimated $6.2 billion in 1978 (Figure 3–1). Federal obligations for health research and development were about $4.1 billion in 1978, or about 66 percent of the total. State and local governments invested $306 million. The remaining $2.1 billion was derived from the private sector: $291 million from private nonprofit agencies and approximately $1.8 billion from industry.

Federal sources of health research support are myriad. Table 3–2 shows the Federal health research budget for 1978, indicating that the Department of Health and Human Services (HHS) controls more than 75 percent of the total, with the National Institutes of Health (NIH) predominant in HHS. NIH alone controls more than two-thirds of the Federal expenditure for health research. This research is largely conducted in universities and medical schools, although NIH has a large in-house research capability.

In the private sector, industry invested almost $1.8 billion in 1978. An estimated $1.3 billion was invested in R&D by the 135 members of the Pharmaceutical Manufacturers Association, which includes some non-drug manufacturers. More than 2,000 firms produce medical devices and instrumentation; these companies invested an estimated $475 million in health R&D. The industry R&D is conducted largely "in-house" in research laboratories, although industry also makes arrangements with outside researchers, including medical academics. Industry also is funded by the Federal government to carry out health R&D. In 1978, NIH obligated about $260 million to industry projects. It is also worth noting that the industry figure has been rising by more than 10 percent a year in recent years, increasing from $1.575 million in 1977 to $1.775 million in 1978 (National Center for Health Statistics, 1980, p. 261).

Basic research is largely funded by the Federal Government, although some is funded by private foundations, voluntary health agencies, and industry. Drug companies invest an estimated $90 million a year in basic research (Silverman and Lee, 1974, p. 14). Other industries spend little on basic research (Mansfield et al., 1971, p. 20). As shown in Table 3–2, about 80 percent of the Federal investment in basic health research comes from NIH.

Applied research is funded by a variety of sources. Much of the support for applied research and technology development is derived from private industry. In fact, most of the industrial R&D budget is spent on applied research and technology development, with priorities usually determined by the perceived potential for profit (Mansfield et al., 1971, p. 20).

Although fragmented and largely undocumented, government invest-

Research and Development 49

Figure 3-1.
Sources of Support for Biomedical R&D in the United States—1978. (millions of dollars)

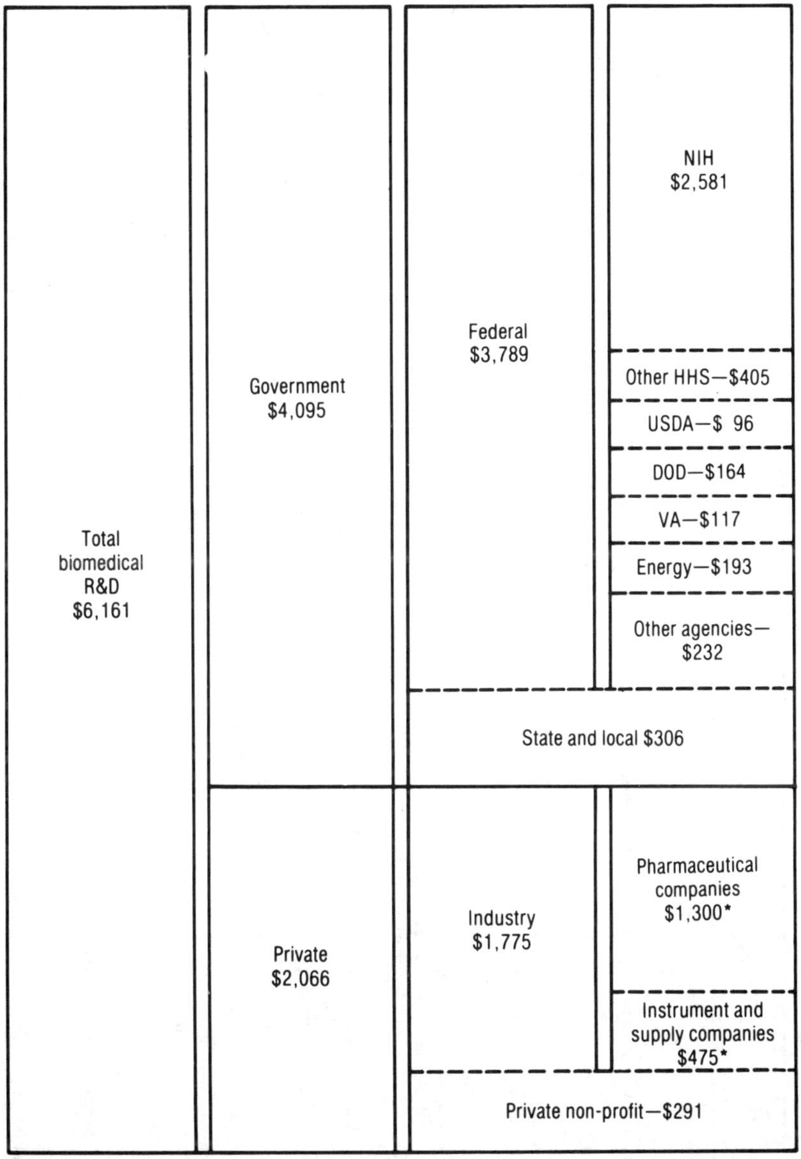

Total biomedical R&D $6,161	Government $4,095	Federal $3,789	NIH $2,581
			Other HHS—$405
			USDA—$ 96
			DOD—$164
			VA—$117
			Energy—$193
			Other agencies—$232
		State and local $306	
	Private $2,066	Industry $1,775	Pharmaceutical companies $1,300*
			Instrument and supply companies $475*
		Private non-profit—$291	

*Estimates
SOURCE: Information compiled by the National Institutes of Health (1979) and the Office of Technology Assessment.

Table 3–2.
Federal Health Research and Development Obligations, By Agency and Estimated Character of Work, Fiscal Year 1978 (In Millions of Dollars)

Agency	Total R & D	Basic research	Applied research	Development
TOTAL FEDERAL	$3,788.8	$1,436.6	$1,912.4	$439.8
Dept. of Health, Education, and Welfare (Total)	2,985.9	1,240.2	1,360.7	385.0
National Institutes of Health (Total)	2,581.3	1,156.0	1,052.6	372.7
Other Public Health Service (Total)	351.4	84.2	255.0	12.2
Alcohol, Drug Abuse, and Mental Health Admin.	180.6	77.5	101.7	1.4
Center for Disease Control	60.1	—	60.1	—
Food and Drug Administration	50.5	—	50.5	—
Health Resources Administration	5.5	—	5.5	—
Health Services Administration	18.4	1.7	9.5	7.2
Office of Asst. Secretary for Health	36.3	5.0	27.7	3.6
Other Dept. of Health, Education, and Welfare (Total)	53.2	—	53.1	0.1
Health Care Financing Administration	19.4	—	19.4	—
Asst. Secretary for Planning and Evaluation	7.7	—	7.7	—
Office of Human Development Services	26.0	—	25.9	0.1
Other Federal Departments and Agencies (Total)	802.9	196.4	551.7	54.8
Department of Agriculture	96.5	35.1	57.2	4.2
Department of Defense	164.4	37.0	113.6	13.8
Department of Energy	193.2	18.0	175.2	—
Department of the Interior	14.4	—	6.7	7.7
Department of State	17.2	—	17.2	—
Environmental Protection Agency	56.6	4.5	52.1	—
National Aeronautics and Space Administration	56.6	28.9	22.9	4.8
National Science Foundation	65.3	62.4	2.9	—
Veterans Administration	117.3	10.0	91.2	16.1
All other Departments and Agencies	21.4	0.5	12.7	8.2

Source: National Institutes of Health, 1979

ment in technology development is also considerable. Research conducted or supported by Federal agencies such as NIH is often aimed directly at the development of new medical technologies. For example, NIH has invested heavily in the development of the totally implantable artificial heart (OTA, 1976, p. 24) and in the possibility of heart transplant. On the other hand, NIH did not invest in the development of CT scanning until after a model built in England was commercially available. Parts of the Federal Government, such as the Veterans Administration and the Department of Commerce, have also encouraged technology development through procurement and incentive programs.

Priority-setting and planning for the support of biomedical research and development are very complex and fragmented. Generally speaking, basic research is funded through "investigator-initiated" research projects, which are reviewed by groups of peers for technical merit. Applied research tends to be done under contract, a situation in which the Federal agency can specify the outcome it seeks.

Problems of Planning Biomedical Research and Development

The mechanisms for support of biomedical R&D have been scrutinized repeatedly during the past ten years (Woldridge, 1965; House of Representatives, 1976a; President's Biomedical Research Panel, 1976; DHEW Health Research Principles, 1978; Brown, 1977; Institute of Medicine, 1979). Each of these reports has raised concerns about the erosion of support for basic biomedical research and has endorsed the importance of such research. The processes used by NIH for funding basic research have consistently been praised. The most recent effort, the DHEW Health Research Principles, stated as its first principle, "A national commitment to fundamental research is essential to meet the full range of public health expectations" (p. 9).

These same reports, however, have identified a number of problems that have not been solved. All of the recent reports have identified weaknesses in the lack of attention given to such areas as epidemiology, economics, statistics, and sociology. In addition, it may be possible to plan applied research activities more effectively to meet the needs of practitioners and Federal programs. This point will be further discussed in Chapter 11.

The present pattern of support for biomedical R&D raises several problems that must be considered if medical technologies under development are to be properly evaluated. First, Federal support for biomedical R&D is administered through a bewildering variety of agencies. Compilation of the budgets and agendas of these agencies, a necessary prerequisite to assessing technologies, is a formidable task in itself. Second, more information about the effects of Federal programs on private investment is needed if the results of evaluation are to be used wisely. Government funds allocated in different ways can encourage, discourage, or displace private investment in R&D (Carter et al., 1976). For example, if assessment of technology results in altered allocations in government service programs, the effects of these changes on industrial expenditures must be anticipated and considered. Finally, most of the targeted development of medical technology currently takes place in the private sector, supported by industry and motivated by the quest for profit (Mansfield et al., 1971, p. 20). Programs of evaluation aimed at Federal agency R&D will necessarily be incomplete, yet assessment of technologies produced by private industry will be difficult, perhaps impossible, to do completely because of lack of access to proprietary information and the resulting ignorance about these developing technologies. Nonetheless, the design and implementation of evaluation processes should take the private activities into account.

4
Adoption of Medical Technologies

> Indeed, what is there that does not appear marvelous when it comes to our knowledge for the first time? How many things, too, are looked upon as quite impossible until they have been actually effected?
>
> Pliny the Elder

The process by which a technology enters and becomes part of the health care system is known as diffusion. It has two phases: the initial period, during which a decision is made within an organization to *adopt* the innovation, and the subsequent and continuing period, encompassing the many decisions to *use* the innovation. Adoption has been studied by researchers far more than use has, and it has been the subject of much greater direct involvement by government. However, as described in Chapter 5, the extent of use of a medical technology can vary considerably. We feel that the degree of imbalance in the literature and government policy on the adoption stage is inadvisable. Government policy has conformed to the traditional noninterference in the decisions of medical practitioners. In so doing, however, it has avoided the search for alternative policies that could provide a reasonable balance between rational technology use and the concern of physicians. Thus, some potential levers for change may have been overlooked.

Diffusion of Some Specific Technologies

As mentioned in Chapter 1, descriptive research has shown that the diffusion process usually describes an S-shaped or sigmoid curve, relating the percentage of potential adopters to actual adopters. It describes what has happened rather than what ought to have happened. Although standards are set down to evaluate adoption, there seems to be a tacit assumption that the adoption of an innovation is desirable. For non-medical technologies that are bought and sold in the marketplace by private firms, whether or not the technology is adopted may be a reasonable test of its desirability. However, the discussion of efficacy and safety in Chapter 6, and of the lack of competition and perverse incentives in the health care system described in Chapter 5, make it clear that, for a medical technology, the act of adoption cannot be considered confirmation of desirability.

Little work has been done on the diffusion of medical technology. Figure 4–1 shows the diffusion of intensive care units in hospitals in the United States. Although the curve has not yet levelled off, it and the following figure (Figure 4–2) for cardiac pacemaker sales are consistent with the classic sigmoid curve. Note that these figures analyze only adoption—not use—a situation typical of this literature.

The diffusion of medical technologies does not always follow the sigmoid curve. One major departure from this model occurs when diffusion reaches a high rate almost immediately after the technology becomes available, as in the case of chemotherapy for leukemia, shown in Figure 4–3.

Figure 4–1.
Diffusion of Intensive Care Units in the United States.

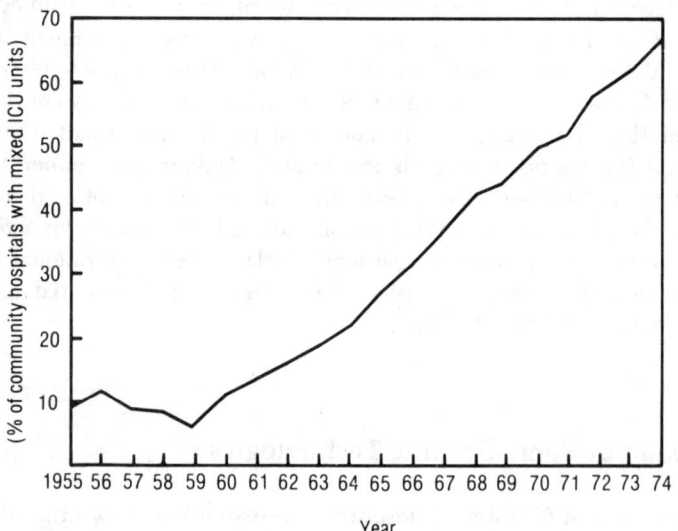

SOURCE: American Hospital Association; redrawn by the Office of Technology Assessment.

Figure 4–2.
Cardiac Pacemaker Sales.

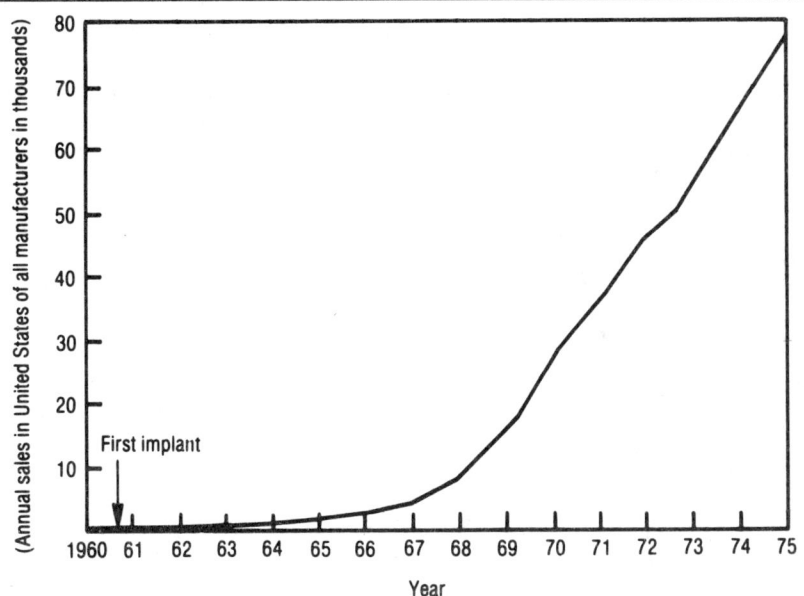

SOURCE: Medtronic, Inc.; redrawn by the Office of Technology Assessment.

This pattern has been referred to as the "desperation-reaction model" (Warner, 1975, 1977). A first phase of rapid diffusion seems to occur because of the provider's sense of responsibility to help the patient and their mutual desperation. Usually, information of efficacy is lacking at this early stage. Somewhat later, results of clinical tests and experience begin to influence the physician's behavior. If results are positive, diffusion may continue rapidly; but if the evidence is not clear-cut, there may be caution and slow diffusion. If the evidence seems negative, use of the technology gradually declines. This points out a paradox in the diffusion of medical technologies. Faced with a desperate situation, each physician may be justified in adopting whatever technology may work. The aggregate behavior of many desperate physicians, however, may result in the extensive and premature diffusion of technologies that are incompletely developed, inefficacious, or possibly even dangerous.

Whatever its initial pattern of diffusion, a technology may be partially or completely abandoned. A number of such examples are mentioned in

Figure 4-3.
Chemotherapy for Children with Leukemia: Connecticut.

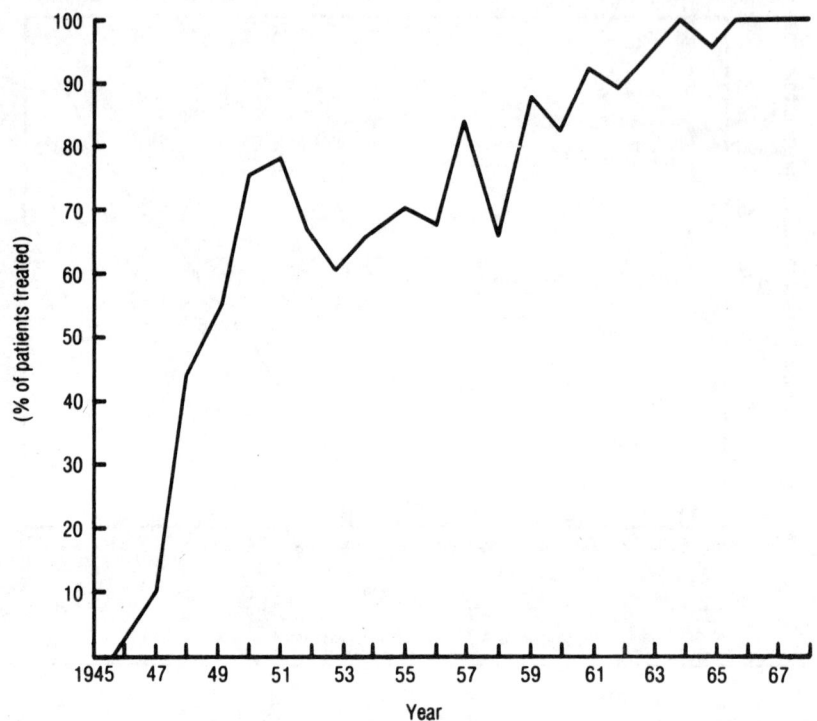

SOURCE: Warner, K. "A 'Desperation-Reaction' Model of Medical Diffusion." *Health Services Research* 10: 369, 1975. Redrawn by the Office of Technology Assessment.

Chapter 6. Figure 4.4 shows a recent example, a psychosurgical procedure known as leucotomy. The same process seems to be occurring now for such surgical procedures as tonsillectomy and radical mastectomy. Such a decrease in utilization can result from additional knowledge or can follow introduction of a more effective technology. That happened with the introduction of polio vaccine, which almost overnight entirely supplanted the costly halfway technology of rehabilitation centers (Thomas, 1974, p. 36).

The following sections will examine the evidence on diffusion more analytically.

Adoption of Medical Technologies

Figure 4-4.
Leucotomy Operations: England and Wales.

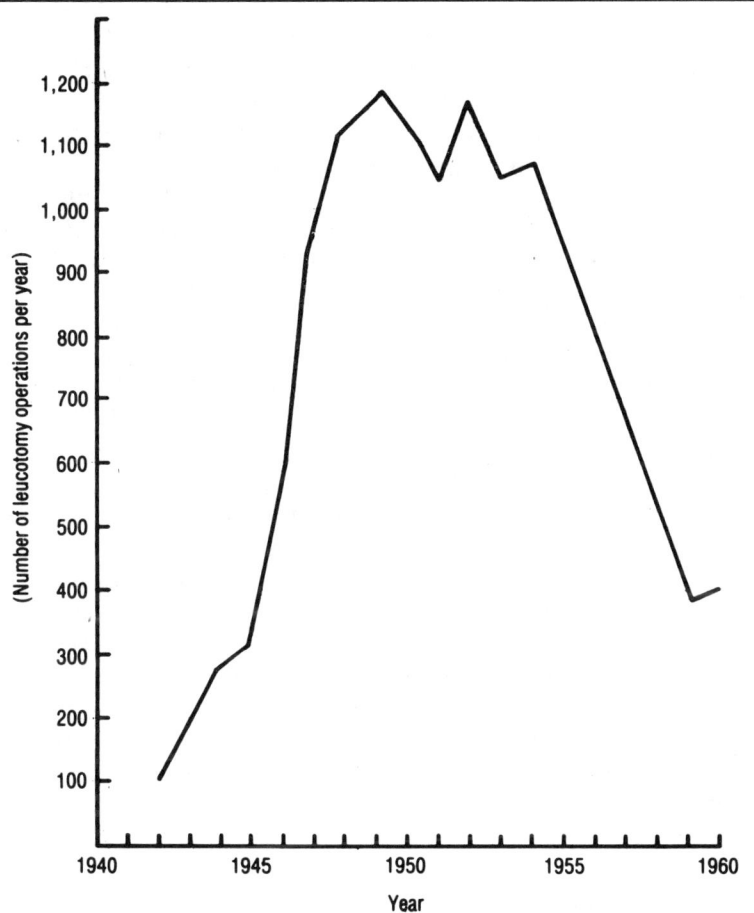

SOURCE: G. Tooth and M. Newton, *Leucotomy in England and Wales 1942-54*, Reports on Public Health and Medical Subjects No. 104 (Ministry of Health, Great Britain: London 1961); redrawn by the Office of Technology Assessment.

Communicating Information About New Technologies

Before adoption or rejection can occur, knowledge about a technology must be communicated to a potential adopter. However, little research has been done on the transferring of information from those who develop it to those who may use it (Young, 1980). In the medical area, only drugs have received the attention of researchers. Industry provides the original source of drug information for physicians (see Chapter 5), although scientific sources become more important in the decision to prescribe (Kaluzny et al., 1975). The research on drugs led to a description of a two-step model, in which information flows initially to physicians who are opinion leaders. Through informal channels, the opinion leaders then transfer information to their followers (Tannon and Rogers, 1975). Such communication among physicians may also explain adoption across organizations.

Considering the problems of efficacy and safety of medical technologies, it is reasonable to be concerned with the premature or inappropriate application of medical innovations prior to clinical evaluation and with the delayed application of useful technologies (Fineberg and Hiatt, 1979; Office of Technology Assessment, 1978a). Besides the problem with evaluation, there is no planned or structured way to channel communication from researchers to practitioners. It has been suggested that scientists, who develop and test innovative medical technologies, hold different norms and values from physicians, who must adopt or reject the technology. The factors that scientists use in evaluating and communicating among themselves are often not attuned to those factors important to clinicians (Young, 1980). Although this transfer of information is poorly understood, little research on the subject is taking place.

Factors Influencing Adoption

Characteristics of Technology

Only the recent literature on technology has begun to question the wisdom of adopting new technologies and has begun to discuss evaluating them (OTA, 1978a, 1978b; Russell, 1979; Committee on Technology and Health Care, 1979).

The earlier literature on adoption focused on characteristics that hastened adoption: relative advantage over previous methods, compatibility with the adopter's values, complexity of understanding and using the innovation, ability to be tested on a limited basis, and observability or visibility of the results to others (Tannon and Rogers, 1975). These characteristics depend on the adopter's perspective and judgment rather than on the nature of the technology. Since adopters' views will vary, confusion about this distinction has been cited as a cause for apparently inconsistent research findings (Downs and Mohr, 1976).

The CT scanner, which was rapidly adopted (see Figure 4–5), exemplifies a technology with many of the characteristics expected to speed adoption (Willems et al., 1979). Compared to its diagnostic alternatives, such as pneumoencephalograms, CT scanning reduced patient discomfort and risk. CT scanning was also financially profitable for providers, an ad-

Figure 4–5.
Cumulative Number of CT Scanners Installed, 1973–1979.

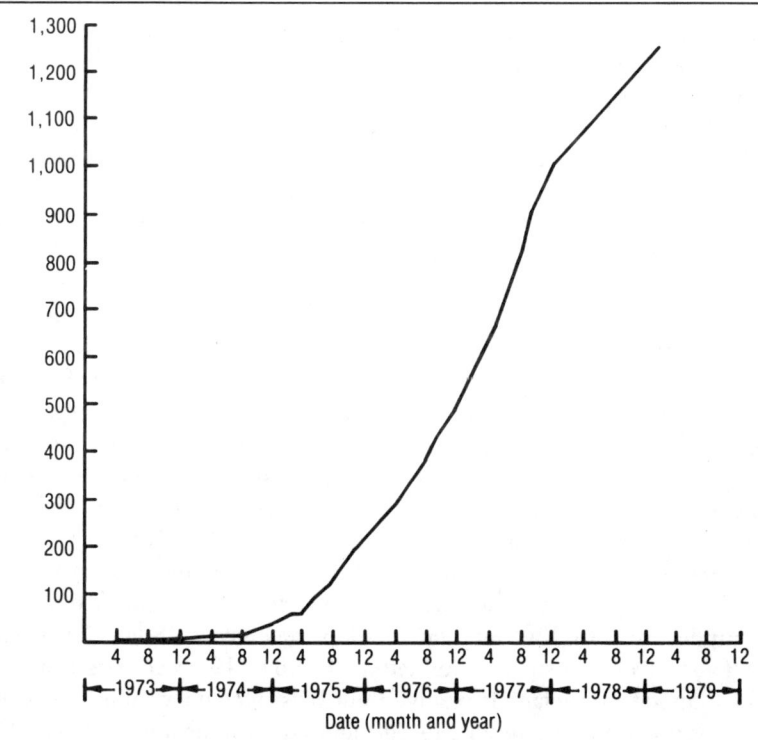

SOURCE: Office of Technology Assessment.

vantage cited by economically oriented studies of adoption. The scanner was compatible with radiology practice, and technicians or physicians needed little additional training. The results of CT examinations were striking because scans visualized hitherto inaccessible portions of the brain. Although the purchase price was about half a million dollars, manufacturers provided initial demonstration models and offered the option of leasing machines.

Characteristics of the Adopter

The adopter of a medical technology, particularly a costly one, is usually an organization, but the literature has mainly centered on individuals, either as practitioners or as actors within institutions. This individual is often referred to as an entrepreneur in the economic literature, and as an opinion leader in the sociological literature.

Studies of individuals have focused on physicians and their use of drugs. Some studies confirm the expectation that physicians with a higher level of training and a higher level of participation in the medical community more readily adopted a new drug, while others have found little association (Tannon and Rogers, 1975). These inconsistent results may be related to the appropriateness of the drugs studied. Some physicians, faced with a drug whose value they doubted, may have rejected or exercised more prudence in adopting it. As noted above, desperation—or availability of alternatives—may also be important.

Within organizations, adoption has generally been associated with members and administrators who had a higher level of training and a more cosmopolitan outlook (Kaluzny et al., 1975; Greer, 1977a). For example, among public health department administrators, early adopters of technologies considered very likely to diffuse, such as measles immunization, were young and cosmopolitan (Kaluzny et al., 1975). In both hospitals and health departments, the administrator's cosmopolitan outlook and the medical staff's educational level were predictors of greater adoption of low-risk innovations, but not of high-risk ones (Kaluzny et al., 1974).

Decisionmaking within organizations is spread among subgroups who have differing interests. The way they reach decisions in the face of conflict has implications for the decision to adopt technology. Some investigators have focused on physician domination (Perrow, 1979). Harris stated that conflict among physicians is resolved not by strategic bargaining, but by an agreement to expand overall capacity and adopt innovations (1977). However, Greer disputed physician domination. She described the hospitals she studied as so uncontrolled that the resolute can accomplish their goals.

She also noted that in her study both administrators and hospital-based physicians promoted new technology to community physicians, who were more resistant to change (1977b). Cromwell et al. (1975) hypothesized that administrators seek sophisticated equipment because it both raises the hospital's prestige and attracts physician specialists to the hospital staff. They found adoption greater in states with more physicians per capita and more specialists per physician.

The structure of an organization has also been examined for its effect on adoption. Greater adoption has been found in acute care hospitals, where the visibility of consequences was high (Kaluzny et al., 1975). Complexity, size, medical school affiliation, and diversity of tasks have all been found to be associated with greater adoption (Greer, 1977a; Rapoport, 1978; Russell, 1976, 1979; Kaluzny et al., 1975; Cromwell et al., 1975). More complex case mix could account for the observation that hospitals associated with medical schools were faster adopters of intensive care units and earlier adopters of radioisotopes (Rapoport, 1978; Russell, 1979). Because size is correlated with several other variables, such as medical school affiliation and financial and personnel resources, the independent effect of each is often unclear. Likewise, conflicting results have been found for centralization of decisionmaking and formalization of procedures (Greer, 1977a; Kaluzny et al., 1975), perhaps because quantifying and measuring such structural variables is very difficult (Tannon and Rogers, 1975).

Kimberly's study of respiratory disease therapies and electronic data processing indicated that Federal hospitals were greater adopters than other kinds of hospitals (1978). This finding may reflect the different case mix and budget procedures in such hospitals. Or, the finding may not be generalizable to other kinds of technologies: Federal hospitals adopted CT scanners more slowly than community hospitals (Banta, 1980b; Willems et al., 1979).

With few exceptions, studies of organizational adoption of medical technologies have been confined to hospitals. Ambulatory care practices, whether solo physicians' offices or group practices, have received little attention. Yet adoption by such practices often accounts for a substantial part of the total. Of the 1254 CT scanners known to be operational in February 1979, 18 percent were located outside of hospitals (OTA, 1980). Although health planning laws exclude ambulatory care practices, they are obviously important and will be more so in the future, as financing encourages ambulatory care services.

Because of economies of scale and vertical integration, group practices have the potential to deliver medical care at lower cost (Fein, 1967; Willems, 1979b). On both organizational and economic grounds, vertical integration may affect technology adoption. Vertical integration is the production by a firm itself of services that would otherwise be provided by the firm's buyers or suppliers (Willems, 1979b). Within health care, a continuum of vertical integration extends from a solo practice with separate diagnostic facilities and hospitals, to ambulatory group practice and separate hospital, to hospital-based group practice, and to community health centers with an even broader range of facilities and services. Under the fragmentation that now characterizes medical care delivery, physicians usually use hospital technologies without cost to themselves. Compared to solo practices or ambulatory groups, a hospital-based group is likely to consider a wider range of costs and benefits when adopting a technology because the integrated group more fully bears the consequences. Decisionmaking would also differ between administrators and physicians and among physician specialties.

The purchase of a CT scanner by Kaiser-Permanente in Northern California suggests that adoption by alternative delivery systems merits examination. In 1976, when Kaiser-Permanente, a hospital-based prepaid group practice, decided to buy a scanner for its 1.3 million members, the state of California already had 60 scanners installed (2.8 per million population) and 119 installed and committed (5.5 scanners per million population) (OTA, 1978b). The group analyzed their situation and purchased a scanner only when the group's use had reached the point at which performing CT scans internally was less costly than buying them externally. Although the contrast with the overall state rate is striking, the group effectively used the technology before purchase of a scanner because it had been obtaining CT scans for its patients from other hospitals. A complete analysis of this case would also consider the younger age of Kaiser members and the capitation payment for service.

Characteristics of the Environment

Those who have studied technology adoption have stressed the importance of conditions external to individual and organizational adopters (Gordon and Fisher, 1975; Committee on Technology and Health Care, 1979; Warner, 1974). These factors are most amenable to manipulation, and include financing methods, market conditions, and government programs. We will describe the policy effects of government programs later in this chapter. However, it should be noted that the financing methods and market conditions also provide a possible avenue for indirect government and other social intervention in adoption, by structuring incentives, creating equivalents for the market, and promoting the development of new institutions (Schultze, 1977).

An important part of the environment that has received little stress in the literature is patient need or demand (White, 1974, 1975). The stress on provider behavior stems in part from the fact that adoption decisions are made primarily by physicians and hospitals. Moreover, good health and the need for care are not precise, objective concepts. Nonetheless, it is remarkable that no striking relationship has emerged between the incidence or prevalence of disease and the adoption of relevant technology. The primary determinant of individual demand for health care appears to be health status (Joseph, 1971). For most technologies studied by Russell (1979), greater hospital adoption occurred in areas of high population growth, a phenomenon related to market expansion. In a study of nonprofit hospitals, Ginsburg (1972) found total investment unresponsive to occupancy rates, taken as an indicator of demand. High occupancy rates did lead to investment in beds, and low rates were associated with other investments. Older hospitals undertook more investment of all kinds, perhaps to replace aging facilities or to stave off decline (Greer, 1977b).

In a broader sense, patient demand for care has a dynamic influence on such factors as the extent and nature of insurance coverage.

FINANCING METHODS. Several economists have attributed increases in medical technologies and medical expenditures to the growth of third-party payment (Feldstein and Taylor, 1977; Russell, 1979). Financing methods and their relation to use will be discussed in Chapter 5. But adoption too is influenced by what is covered by insurance and the methods of payment used. Adoption of expensive hospital technologies is fostered because third parties pay more than 90 percent of all hospital expenditures (National Center for Health Statistics, 1978, Table 162). On the other hand, the much less complete coverage of preventive, rehabilitative, and ambulatory services inhibits their adoption.

Medicare as well as some Blue Cross/Blue Shield plans reimburse hospitals and other institutional providers on the basis of the actual costs that they have incurred in the course of delivering services. Fee-for-service payment for charges billed is the typical method for reimbursing physicians. Usually, in the markets for goods and services, financial payment has a deterrent effect; it forces those demanding services to make trade-offs between more units and more funds. However, health insurance as presently constituted removes or lessens the financial restraints that would otherwise restrict technology adoption. Third-party payments generally cover the expenses of new technology whether they are for the purchase, maintenance, or operation of equipment; the leasing of equipment; the cost of drugs; or the facilities and equipment needed for a procedure. Physicians' inclination to rely on medical technology may stem from their medical training and professional socialization (see Chapter 5), but current insurance methods facilitate that reliance. And certain technologies prove quite lucrative. Estimates of the annual profit from a CT head scanner in 1976 ranged from about $50,000 to $300,000, or from 11 to 65 percent of the purchase price per year (OTA, 1978b). This is not only a problem for "big" technology. Showstack and Schroeder (1979) estimated that a gastroscopy costs the physician about $41, but that the fee for the procedure averages $240.

Some studies have found that third-party payment has stimulated technology adoption. Comparing different states, Cromwell and his associates (1975) found that the percentage of revenues from third parties was significantly and positively related to hospital adoption of expensive technology. Russell reported that the adoption of cobalt therapy and electroencephalography occurred more quickly where the level of insurance coverage was higher, and proceeded more rapidly as the level grew. As Medicare's contribution to a hospital's total costs rose, so did the adoption of cobalt, intensive care beds, and diagnostic radioisotopes. Open heart surgery was adopted more quickly in areas where insurance coverage was growing faster (Russell, 1979).

In light of the stimulus to indiscriminant technology adoption provided by prevailing financing methods, prospective reimbursement has been advanced as an alternative, whereby rates are set prior to the period during which they apply. Forms of prospective reimbursement vary according to the unit of payment (service, case, consumer, institutional, or provider budget), the mechanism for setting and adjusting rates, and the disposition of any surpluses or deficits at the end of the period. Like all payment methods, the different prospective reimbursement arrangements would be expected to have different effects on provider revenues and on technology adoption. A research project currently underway is investigating the effect of different forms of prospective reimbursement on the adoption of specific technologies (Wagner, 1978).

AVAILABILITY OF FINANCIAL CAPITAL. The purchase of medical equipment or the construction of facilities for medical technology clearly constitutes investment and requires funds. Aspects of capital availability include access to funds and the terms of funding, such as interest rates and payback periods. The availability of capital could limit the amount of technology that a potential adopter would purchase, or an adopter's choice among specific technologies. However, the sensitivity of medical adopters to the availability of external sources of financial capital is not clear.

Third-party payments affect internal and external sources. Medicare, for example, reimburses institutional providers for capital as well as operating costs. Medicare payment for allowable capital costs such as depreciation and interest provides a source of internally generated funds. But depreciation is on a historical rather than a replacement cost basis, and with recent inflation rates, accumulated depreciation falls short of the amount needed for replacement. Also, Medicare will not pay for any accumulated reserves or for bad debts of other patients (Bice et al., 1976).

Third-party coverage, especially Medicare for the elderly and Medicaid for the poor, has reduced hospitals' risk of bad debts. Along with secure sources of operating expenses, third-party payment has thereby improved hospitals' standing as credit risks to private lenders.

Other changes in governmental programs have affected sources of financial capital. The Hill-Burton program funded construction and modernization of medical care facilities. Federal governmental grants under the Hill-Burton program have declined since 1970 (Russell and Burke, 1975). The program will be described later in this chapter.

As cost reimbursement applied to capital costs and made hospitals better financial risks, Federal and state laws facilitated borrowing through tax-exempt bonds. In 1976, 46 states had public corporations authorized to issue such bonds for hospitals (Gelfand, 1978).

Since the 1960s, hospitals have continually increased their reliance on debt financing as a source of funds (Ginsburg, 1972). Illustrative of this trend, community hospitals drew 31 percent of their funds for construction from debt financing in 1966, but 64 percent in 1975 (Gelfand, 1978; Manley and Ashley, 1977). This represented a shift away from primarily governmental and secondarily philanthropic and internal sources. Within the category of debt financing for construction in 1975, tax-exempt bond issues provided 56 percent of community hospital funds and 68 percent of governmental hospital funds. Investor-owned hospitals relied primarily on commercial loans, which accounted for 45 percent of their construction funds.

Of particular interest for technology adoption, one marketing analysis designated tax-exempt bonds and leases as the major financing vehicles to secure major equipment (Kelling and Williams, 1976). The analysis considered bond funds the major purchasers of tax-exempt bonds, and commercial banks the major source of funds for leases.

MARKET STRUCTURE. General agreement exists that any competition among medical care providers typically is not based on price (Russell, 1979). Since the price of technology has little effect on providers and patients under existing insurance, one would expect greater adoption of technology to occur than under more price competition. Even for the diffusion of nonmedical technologies, the degree of competition and the extent of innovation have not shown a clear relationship (Kennedy and

Thirlwell, 1972). Innovation may thrive most in intermediate degrees of competition rather than in extremes (Kamien, 1975).

Studies of hospitals have found no definite relationship between measures of competition and adoption. The situation is complex, because the characteristics of the market may relate not only to competitiveness, but also to the availability and sharing of information and to local standards of practice. The evidence conflicts, depending on the characteristic used and the technology studied. Russell (1979) found that concentration of market power among a few large hospitals did not appear to influence the adoption of three common and two prestige technologies, but that hospitals in more concentrated markets were less likely to adopt open heart surgery. Prior adoption in a locality reportedly speeded the adoption of intensive care units and electroencephalographs, but not diagnostic radioisotopes, open heart surgery, renal dialysis, cobalt therapy, and computers (Cromwell et al., 1975; Russell, 1979). In urban areas, greater adoption of radioisotopes and electronic data processing occurred where there were many hospitals per capita, the hospitals were of similar size, and they were close to other hospitals (Kimberly, 1978; Rapoport, 1978).

Different patterns have also been observed between adoption and the number of physicians per capita. Facing a low physician–population ratio, hospitals may compete for physicians through technology adoption. On the other hand, fewer physicians may exert less pressure for adoption. The adoption of CT scanners and radioisotopes appeared unrelated to the physician-population ratio (Rapoport, 1978; Willems et al., 1979). However, greater adoption of intensive care units, open heart surgery, cobalt therapy, and renal dialysis occurred among states with higher ratios (Cromwell et al., 1975).

Federal Activities to Influence Adoption

A number of Federal programs have developed whose aim is to influence adoption. Some have been aimed at speeding adoption. Others have been aimed at channeling adoption, either through providing information or requiring careful evaluation before adoption is allowed. Programs to evaluate medical technologies and programs regulating efficacy and safety of technologies are described in Chapter 6. This section will describe other programs.

It should be noted that the literature on diffusion contains little evaluation of the effects of policy interventions on adoption, which is surprising, since those factors are more amenable to manipulation than such factors as the nature of institutions and adopters. This is a research gap that needs to be addressed (Willems, 1979b).

Programs to Facilitate Adoption

From 1965 to 1975, the Regional Medical Program (RMP) disseminated information about new technologies and gave grants to speed their adoption. It resulted from the belief that aggressive diffusion of technology would improve health. Although now defunct, RMP is instructive as a government program that successfully promoted adoption. The program initially concentrated on heart disease, cancer, and stroke, then added kidney disease in 1970. Russell (1979) concluded that RMP stimulated the adoption of intensive care units as a means of treating heart attacks and strokes. She detected no effect on renal dialysis, however.

Another program aimed at promoting the adoption of technology is the National Blood Pressure Education Program, based at the National Institutes of Health. The program is a modestly funded attempt to increase public and professional awareness of the importance of high blood pressure as a health problem. The program has supported mass media campaigns, school health programs, and attempts to reach physicians. Although no definitive evaluation of the program has been conducted, the number of people in the United States effectively treated rose dramatically during the 1970s.

Finally, the Hill-Burton program was developed as an attempt to promote technology—that is, hospital beds. The program began in 1946 to stimulate the construction of new hospitals, nursing homes, rehabilitation centers, and other health facilities, emphasizing rural areas and other areas where facilities were scarce. Under the law, each state was required to have a planning agency that established a statewide plan for construction projects. This was the beginning of state planning in the health facility field. The program was both popular and successful. After 1970, it began to emphasize urban areas and ambulatory care facilities. However, in 1973, the administration concluded that the nation had too many general hospitals, and the program was essentially abolished in 1974 legislation (Miles, 1974, pp. 211–212).

Programs for Acquiring Technology by Government Agencies

A number of special government committees give advice on specific technologies. A notable example is the Immunization Practices Advisory Committee (IPAC). It advises the Centers for Disease Control (CDC) about government policy towards immunization, including which vaccines to provide in Federal campaigns. Consisting of clinicians and state public health officials, IPAC bases its recommendations on data provided by the Food and Drug Administration and CDC about the safety and efficacy of a vaccine and about the etiology, natural history, and epidemiology of the disease.

Activities of the Veterans Administration (VA) affect adoption of technologies within the VA Medical Centers and by others as well. The Supply Service of the VA tests and evaluates new equipment for safety and technical performance, and other organizations, such as the Public Health Service Hospitals, refer to the VA supply catalogue in making procurement decisions. The Supply Service evaluated several models of CT scanners before adoption. When the VA purchased three body scanners in 1977, it solicited bids from the known manufacturers and accepted a bid substantially below the usual price per scanner, $375,000 compared to $450,000 (OTA, 1978b).

Under the VA's program of Specialized Medical Services, technologies are centrally evaluated and approved for acquisition on the basis of safety, effectiveness, and costs. Currently applicable to about 50 services, this program was designed to rationalize the adoption of technologies for major medical problems of VA patients. Examples of included services are alcohol dependence treatment centers, intensive care units, and spinal cord injury centers. The VA is in the process of devising a procedure for evaluation of other technologies before their adoption by VA Medical Centers. VA activities relating to adoption extend beyond the VA system. More than 90 of its Medical Centers have agreements to share specialized facilities, such as renal dialysis centers, with community providers.

The Federal Health Resources Sharing Committee, representing such agencies as the VA, HHS (Health and Human Services), and the Department of Defense, has begun to coordinate on issues of expensive specialized technologies. The Committee initially explored the closure of facilities, such as a VA cardiac catheterization laboratory, but may also coordinate decisions to adopt and place technologies. Subcommittees have been established for CT scanners, health information systems, and cancer treatment.

The Health Planning Program

Although the health planning laws require a number of activities related to planning for technologies, the major power of these programs is in regulating capital investment by private institutions.

REGULATION OF CAPITAL INVESTMENT. The power to regulate capital investment rests on three overlapping programs: Section 1122 review, state certificate-of-need laws, and the National Health Planning and Resources Development Act. Since 1972, Section 1122 of the Social Security Act has allowed the Medicare and Medicaid programs to withhold funding for depreciation, interest, and return on equity capital for certain investments found inconsistent with a state health plan. The provision applied to investments of more than $100,000. Section 1122 covers changes in beds and services that are provided by certain health care facilities, such as hospitals, skilled nursing facilities, kidney disease treatment centers, and ambulatory surgical facilities. Although Health Maintenance Organizations (HMOs) are included, private physicians' offices are explicitly exempted. In 1977, 37 states had contracted with the Department of Health and Human Services to conduct Section 1122 reviews.

State certificate-of-need (CON) laws in effect constitute a franchising process for potential adopters of expensive medical technologies. Enacted by 35 states by 1977, these laws require prior approval by the state of investments above a certain threshold, usually $100,000 or more. Although the laws vary, most apply to hospitals and nursing homes and to bed construction. Like Section 1122, most CON laws exempt private physicians. Sanctions include denial of operating licenses, court injunctions, and fines.

The National Health Planning and Resources Development Act of 1974 required states to pass CON laws as a condition of future Federal funding under the Public Health Service Act, the Community Mental Health Centers Act, and the Alcohol Abuse and Alcoholism Act. The Planning Act applied to the same facilities covered by Section 1122 review. However, the 1979 Planning Act amendments exempted HMOs from securing a certificate-of-need for inpatient investments because of a belief in the efficiency of such plans. The Planning Act stipulates that CON laws apply to capital expenditures of at least $150,000 and higher, a threshold higher than that for Section 1122 review.

THE PROCESS OF REGULATING CAPITAL INVESTMENT. Local Health Systems Agencies (HSAs) have responsibility for areawide planning and initial CON review. At the state level, the State Health Planning and Development Agency (SHPDA) administers the state certificate-of-need programs and assists the Statewide Health Coordinating Council (SHCC) in coordinating planning. The SHPDA is also the State Agency for Section 1122 review. In reviewing CON applications, the agencies are to consider such factors as the population's need for services, the availability of necessary resources, and the effect of construction projects on the applicant's costs of providing services.

In 1978, the National Guidelines for Health Planning, required under the 1974 Act, set quantitative standards for several specific technologies: general hospital beds, obstetrical inpatient services, neonatal special care units, pediatric inpatient services, open heart surgery, cardiac catheterization, and end-stage renal disease services. These standards were to be used for the development of area and state plans required under the 1974 Act (Department of HEW, 1978a).

The Guidelines contain a mixture of standards. Some are based on numbers by population (less than four non-Federal, short-stay hospital beds per 1000 population). Others set minimums (a minimum of 20 pediatric inpatient services beds in units in urban areas). Finally, some of the Guidelines require certain minimum levels of use for existing units of a technology in an area before a provider may add a new unit. For example, no new megavoltage radiation therapy units should be approved unless the existing unit(s) is performing at least 6000 treatments per year. The standards will evolve and change. For example, the draft 1978 Guidelines called for existing CT scanners in an HSA area to be performing 2500 procedures annually before additional scanners received approval. In 1979, the final Guidelines permitted relaxing the standard for such factors as the time required to perform different types of scans and local conditions related to distance, specialized facilities, and labor practices.

EVALUATION OF CAPITAL INVESTMENT REGULATION. The effect of Section 1122 review is controversial. Since the statute excludes operating expenses and physicians' services, only a small percentage of a provider's total revenue may be at risk of scrutiny or control. For example, the operating expenses of CT scanners account for as much as 50 to 75 percent of its technical expenses (OTA, 1978b). Although analysts agree that compliance is widespread, they differ in attributing it to the potential threat of stronger regulation and providers' tradition of being law abiding (Lewin and Associates, 1975) or the slight inconvenience posed by the procedure (OTA, 1978b).

In an early study of certificate-of-need laws, Salkever and Bice (1976, 1979) reported reduced hospital expenditures on beds, but unchanged overall hospital investment. Faced with greater control over beds, hospitals may have channeled their investments to other technologies. Furthermore, as Ginsburg (1972) had found earlier, occupancy was positively associated with bed expansion, although occupancy rates had no apparent effect on total hospital investment.

Cromwell et al. (1975) investigated the effect of certificate-of-need laws on adoption of specific technologies. CON appeared to reduce adoption rates for expensive, widely adopted technologies—namely x-rays and cobalt and radium therapies—but did not affect other technologies examined.

The existence of planning legislation was not correlated with interstate differences in the adoption of CT scanners (Willems et al., 1979). In fact, impending legislation may have spurred adoption as providers rushed to place orders before the law applied to CT scanners. Such an effect may have occurred in California, for example, whose 1976 law exempted equipment already ordered (Banta, 1980a).

PROGRAM DEFICIENCIES. The 1979 Planning Amendments perpetuate a problem in the 1974 law—the exclusion of private physicians' offices from review. At the end of 1977, the laws of only seven states covered physicians' offices. This exclusion has the effect of treating the technology differently, depending on its setting or ownership (OTA, 1978b). Some technologies may lend themselves to placement in private offices, and such placement permits circumvention of the CON process. For example, in 1979 about 18 percent of all CT scanners known to be operational were installed outside of hospitals (OTA, 1980). In addition, a substantial number of scanners were located in hospitals but were exempt from review because they were owned or leased by physicians (Willems et al., 1979).

The case of CT scanning illustrated another generic problem faced by planners: the lack of information about the need for or efficacy of a technology (Banta and Sanes, 1978b). Under the 1974 legislation, planners are to consider need, a difficult subjective concept at best. Chapter 6 describes the evaluation of efficacy and safety. For CT scanners, as for many other medical technologies, scant information about efficacy existed when planners began to receive certificate-of-need applications. Although technical centers are beginning to develop some information for planners, the medical community continues to suffer a general deficiency of evaluations and syntheses about clinical applications that could aid decisionmaking.

Financing Programs and Adoption

Payment for services obviously affects adoption of technology. Methods of payment and third-party coverage will be discussed in more detail in the next chapter. This section will focus on attempts by formal programs to influence adoption through reimbursement policies.

DECISIONS TO COVER SPECIFIC TECHNOLOGIES. The decision of whether or not to include coverage for a specific service in the insurance benefit package is assumed to have a major influence on adoption. The Social Security Act restricts payment in the Medicare and Medicaid programs to those services that are "reasonable and necessary" for diagnosis, treatment, or improved functioning. The Health Care Financing Administration (HCFA) has taken primarily a passive posture, reacting once coverage questions have been raised, usually by the carriers that administer the Medicare program. Over time, different Public Health Service agencies have performed the function of advising Medicare on coverage decisions. The advice has usually been asked only when the technology is controversial. This function now resides, by statute, in the new National Center for Health Care Technology (NCHCT).

Four criteria have been used in evaluating technologies for coverage: safety, efficacy, acceptance by providers, and stage of development (OTA, 1978b). For drugs, Medicare has limited coverage to indications for use that the Food and Drug Administration has approved for labeling. Evaluations of other technologies have been informal and nonsystematic. Staff of the evaluating PHS agency contacted Federal agencies, professional associations, and others for their judgments. If available, formal studies were also used. NCHCT has established a procedure for gaining advice from relevant parts of the National Institutes of Health. Also under consideration is expansion of the criteria to include relative efficacy and cost-effectiveness when considering alternative technologies (Cleeman, 1979). NCHCT is also coordinating its activities with other bodies. It is working with HCFA and certain private third-party payers to evaluate angioplasty (a procedure to dilate plugged coronary arteries), with the Food and Drug Administration on reagent kits to measure alpha-fetoprotein in maternal serum, and with NIH to include economic analyses in Consensus Development Conferences.

Until the case of CT scanning, Medicare's refusal to cover technologies had generally been limited to those that were clearly outmoded or useless. In 1973 Medicare refused to reimburse for CT scans on the grounds that CT scanning had not been established to be reasonable and necessary. Reimbursement for CT head scans on certain machines was subsequently approved. In 1978 reimbursement for body scanning was approved for certain medical conditions. The issue of CT scanning represented a new direction in reimbursement policy. Medicare withheld coverage of a widely hailed technology pending evaluation of its efficacy. Medicare also considered fee levels in evaluating body scans. The precedent of consideration of efficacy is likely to be followed in the future. It is worth noting that these "go slow" decisions did not seem to have any significant effect on the rapid adoption of CT scanners.

Blue Cross and Blue Shield plans have taken similar steps to link reimbursement with efficacy. Until 1977, for example, the national Blue Shield organization advised against reimbursement for CT body scanning on the grounds that data about its efficacy were insufficient. With the advice of specialty societies, Blue Shield has compiled a list of procedures for which they will pay only if physicians justify medical necessity.

Linkages Between Health Planning and Reimbursement

Some Blue Cross/Blue Shield plans have a policy making conformity with planning procedures a general condition of payment. In 1976 about 70 percent of Blue Cross plans responding to a survey either had conformance clauses in their contracts or operated in states with certificate-of-need laws. There have also been some similar but not so widespread activities by commercial insurers (OTA, 1978b). Because of the nature of Section 1122, the Medicare and Medicaid programs do not require full conformity with planning procedures as a condition of payment. The possibility of changing that situation is being explored by HCFA.

HCFA has applied a conformance requirement on mobile CT scanners. Although mobile units may cost less than $100,000 or $150,000 (the typical planning thresholds) they are subject to planning requirements because they represent a substantial change in services offered. The extent to which this decision affects adoption will depend on the degree of leverage exerted by Medicare payment on providers and patients.

Discussion

The linkages between planning and financing, and the possible use of scientific evaluations in these processes, deserve much more attention from researchers and policymakers. While it is clear that the complexities are enormous, rational public policy demands attention to these factors. While there are political problems, it appears that the future lies in this direction.

5
Factors Affecting Use of Technology by Providers

> There are no villains in the piece . . . It is what normal men and women find that they must and will do in spite of their intentions, that really concern us.
>
> George Bernard Shaw

Use of technology is an aspect of diffusion that has received little attention in the medical literature and in the formulation of policy. Attention has focused almost entirely on the adoption stage. That is ironic, of course, since it is the use of technology that is of most concern.

No general relationship has been established between the existence or adoption of a technology and its use. It has been found that hospital beds tend to be filled regardless of health problems or the nature of an area (Roemer and Shain, 1959). It appears that the ready availability of clinical laboratory tests has stimulated a rapid increase in the number of laboratory tests done (OTA, 1976, p. 10). Although availability may increase use, the extent of use generated is not clear for many technologies. Cromwell and his colleagues (1975), for example, reported that nonprofit hospitals in Massachusetts used certain diagnostic equipment at only 50 to 60 percent of capacity. Available evidence in late 1979 indicated that operational CT scanners were being used considerably under capacity (OTA, 1980).

Chapter 7 will analyze measures of evaluating costs of medical technologies. Obviously, costs and use of technology are related. Greater use of a specific medical technology may lower the per unit cost of a service as providers gain more experience or as fixed costs are spread over a greater volume of output. However, greater use may raise total costs as the technology is applied in circumstances where it has little efficacy or where it duplicates other technologies (OTA, 1976). For example, automation of the clinical laboratory has driven unit costs to very low levels. But proliferation of aggregate clinical laboratory testing and increasing expenditures for health care have also resulted.

Although the medical community is basically conservative about incorporating new developments into routine practice, certain factors have encouraged greater use of technologies, however marginal their efficacy. Other factors tend to discourage the use of certain technologies. This chapter discusses some of these dynamic behavioral factors, including professionalism, specialization of physicians, malpractice, organization of practice, and payment for services.

Patient Needs and Technology

It goes almost without saying that medical technology is directed to the solution of human problems. The patient visits a physician seeking advice or help, impelled by a symptom or concern. Quite often the patient has physical disease. After making a diagnosis, the physician may prescribe a therapy—a technology. Thus, the relation between human needs and the use of technology is obvious.

What is surprising is not that technology is addressed to needs, but that so much use of technology appears to be discretionary. Chapter 6 points out the importance of defining the medical problem to be addressed and the patient population involved before it is possible to state whether a technology is efficacious. It is discretionary use—and overuse—that makes this a critical part of the definition of efficacy.

Even for clearly defined technologies addressed to clear-cut medical conditions, use varies remarkably. Wennberg and Gittelsohn (1973) have studied the rates of use of common surgical procedures such as tonsillectomy, hysterectomy, and appendectomy in New England, and have found that rates of tonsillectomy varied from 20 per thousand to 5.6 per thousand depending on area of the country (House of Representatives, 1975, 1976b). The same study examined rates of tonsillectomy among Medicaid-eligible patients and found rates varying from 1709 per 100,000 in Nevada, to 179 per 100,000 in Arkansas. In 1968 Federal employees who received medical care from 14 prepaid group practice plans underwent appendectomy at the rate of 110 per 100,000, while Federal employees enrolled in Blue Shield underwent appendectomy at the rate of 210 per 100,000 (Perrott, 1971). The rates of hysterectomy among Medicaid-eligibles varied from 34 per 100,000 in Mississippi, to 2488 in Nevada (House of Representatives, 1975). Although a part of these differences could be explained by health needs, it is inconceivable that differences of such magnitude could be so explained.

The Physician and Technology

Professionalism and Technology

Physicians are professionals who have a high degree of autonomy. We usually think of professionalism as a way of assuring the quality of services. However, professionalism has other important implications. "Control by an occupational group over its technology is what basically distinguishes a profession from other groups" (Smith and Kaluzny, 1975, p. 161). Or, as Friedson said:

> Arguing from his conceded expertise in diagnosis and treatment, [the physician] is well equipped to influence if not control many other areas of his work. Only a fellow professional may say no, for counterargument can be justified only by reference to knowledge of the special characteristics of the work. Autonomy over the technical character of his work, then, gives him the wherewithal by which to be a 'free' professional, even though he is dependent upon the state for establishing and sustaining his autonomy [Friedson, 1970, p. 46].

The expenditures on health care that result from physicians' services are far greater than the direct costs of the physicians' services. Physicians play a central role in determining the nature and content of medical practice: they decide, for example, who will be admitted to hospitals, how long the patients will stay, what tests will be performed, and what drugs will be prescribed. Thus, physicians' decisions result in expenditures far beyond the direct billings of those physicians. It has been estimated, based on data from the early 1970s, that the average total expenditure obligated per physician exceeds $250,000 (Reinhardt, 1977). More recent data indicate that it may exceed $400,000 (Doty, 1980).

All groups of health workers are now seeking to emulate physicians in creating the same bureaucratic immunity that physicians have (Smith and Kaluzny, 1975, p. 164). The autonomy of physicians explains, for example, why quality assurance mechanisms such as PSROs (see Chapter 9) are controlled by or composed of physicians.

Traditionally, the physician acts as the agent of the patient. The physician's role is to defend the interest of the patient against any other competing interest (Mechanic, 1977). This "social contract" binds physicians to provide the best possible care—apparently regardless of cost (Arrow, 1963). In a climate of full insurance coverage, where the cost to the patient of a procedure is small, the physician has little reason not to use technology if there is a possibility of benefit. Furthermore, possession of modern equipment can increase a physician's income and enhance prestige.

Influence of physicians over the system of health care is even greater than implied by their professional autonomy, however. Physicians have high prestige and tend to be deferred to. They act politically as a group to maintain and retain their prerogatives. The majority of boards of Blue Shield Organizations are controlled by physicians (Delbanco et al., 1979). Physicians tend to control the credentialing of other health workers. And since nearly everyone is sick at one time or the other, most people have reason to be grateful to a skillful and sympathetic physician.

In recent years, physicians have become increasingly bureaucratized through group and institutional practice (Mechanic, 1977). While in part this is a rational response to the growing complexity of medical care, it has wider implications, as discussed in a later section.

Specialization and Technology

The growth in medical specialities is one of the most important phenomena of medical care and one that has tremendous implications for the use of technology. By 1976 only 39 percent of all active U.S. physicians were in primary care specialities of general and family practice, internal medicine, and pediatrics (GMENAC, 1979). In both medicine and surgery, new specialities and subspecialities continue to develop and grow. In part, specialization has been the result of technology. But the growth of specialities has been molded historically more by professional and economic interests than as a response to real needs (Stevens, 1971). Mechanic estimates that a relatively small proportion of physicians—perhaps 15 or 20 percent—could meet the need for consulting specialities (1974, p. 48).

The relationship between greater specialization and technology use is complex and multidirectional (Committee on Technology and Health Care, 1979). The development of new technologies has often spawned new specialities: radiology from x-ray, nuclear medicine from radioisotopes, and vascular surgery from techniques including implantation of blood vessels and replacement of vessels with grafts. Residency positions in the new speciality also are created to train physicians to use the new technologies and to provide services to patients in hospitals that provide the new specialized services. But the very presence of a cadre of specialists may stimulate the use of their services as they exercise their skill and as other physicians refer patients. To earn their incomes, physicians pursue their practice, and in so doing attract sophisticated equipment and its accompanying manpower.

To the extent that specialization improves the quality of care, this expenditure may well be appropriate. Misgivings have arisen, however, about the orientation of medical training and the numbers of specialists trained. As mentioned in Chapter 2, medical education now depends on hospital-based clinical training dominated by a full-time faculty of specialists. Medical education entails the socialization of those entering the medical profession to that model. Students are oriented to rely on and to use the specialized technologies housed in a teaching hospital and to pursue specialty practice, with its higher prestige and income, rather than primary care (Jonas, 1978).

> Physicians are trained to believe that they cannot practice medicine without a hospital close by, a variety of specialized facilities and personnel, and the various components of a highly specialized division of labor. Having been trained primarily within a hospital context, they have become unfitted to perform the more ordinary and mundane tasks that many patients need and want. . . . Moreover, the nature of the division of labor itself, with its dependence on referrals, and the use of various specialized personnel, cause even the most simple of medical services to become extremely expensive [Mechanic, 1972, p. 35].

The actual effect of this orientation may be more complex. One study found that physicians trained in medical schools and hospitals that stress teaching and research rather than practice exhibited more flexibility in adjusting the use of technical services, such as x-ray and laboratory tests, to the needs of the patient (Pineault, 1977). Compared to other physicians, they used fewer technical services when ambiguity about diagnosis was low, such as for chronic and acute disease, but more technical services under greater uncertainity, such as for undiagnosed conditions. It may be that more scientifically oriented medical schools teach their students how to apply technologies selectively. However, other studies have found no relationship between lab use and medical school (Schroeder et al., 1973). In a study of Kaiser-Permanente physicians, no relationship was found between lab use and residency training, but the results may not be generalizable to other practice settings or to other graduates of those medical schools. In the Kaiser-Permanente system, physicians in leadership positions have lower lab use, a style of practice that other physicians in the organization may emulate (Freeborn et al., 1972).

It is also possible that greater specialization can follow from an excess supply of physicians. Physicians may enter specialty practice and use specialized technologies as a response to a glut in the market for physician services (Evans, 1976). Prevailing payment methods facilitate if not encourage this trend, as discussed later. This possibility is of great importance, since the United States is facing a possible excess of physicians. As Reinhardt points out, it is not necessary to behave in bad conscience, but only to recognize the extent of discretionary use possible. "Surely there must be enough tests, revisits for chronic conditions, check-ups or muscular-skeletal reconstructions that are of some benefit to patients . . . especially when time is available to do so and no fiscal hardship is thereby visited directly on the individual patient" (1977).

Empirical studies to demonstrate that specialists use more medical technologies have produced contradictory results. To a certain extent, the answer is obvious. For those specialities that are dependent on a particular technology, increased use must be so. For technologies not associated closely with a particular specialty group, several studies have not confirmed greater technology use by specialists than by nonspecialists (Freeborn et al., 1972; Pineault, 1976; Schroeder et al., 1973). One study reported greater x-ray use by specialists, but did not adjust for case mix or severity (Childs and Hunter, 1972). Another study found that different specialists use technology differently (Wagner et al., 1976). Russell (1979, p. 161) found in a nationwide study that areas with more surgeons adopted cobalt therapy and open heart surgery more frequently than other areas.

The consistent finding that physicians use diagnostic technologies at lower rates the longer they have been practicing suggests a learning curve. Over time physicians may gain experience and confidence. However, any such cycle still occurs within the secular trend of greater use of diagnostic and other technologies by the medical profession.

Although not thoroughly analyzed here, the orientation of medical education and the numbers and types of specialists trained are issues amenable to influence and direction from both public and private quarters. The Graduate Medical Education National Advisory Committee (GMENAC, 1979), as charged by Federal legislation, consists of public and private representatives who are considering these very issues. Similarly, a report by the Institute of Medicine, which incorporated a wide range of views, suggested altering the number and types of physicians trained. That report alluded to, but did not explicitly analyze, the interrelationship between specialization and technology use (Committee on Technology and Health Care, 1979).

In summary, most indications are that specialization is associated with increasing use of technology. A specialty is generally involved with a specific technology (or technologies) that it believes in and wants to apply. When associated with a payment system that rewards specialty services highly, and a public that generally is satisfied with our present specialty-oriented system (American Medical Association, 1978; Health Insurance Institute, 1979), it seems likely that specialization is a key factor influencing the use of technology.

Liability for Malpractice

By the mid-1970s, malpractice litigation had become a major concern in the United States. Providers' apprehensions about malpractice suits have frequently been cited to explain technology use (Committee on Technology and Health Care, 1979). Once the use of a technology becomes part of "accepted medical practice," physicians and hospitals may feel compelled to provide it to patients. Few reports or empirical studies, though, have linked lack of use of technology to malpractice. Fear of malpractice has been cited as a reason for the overuse of skull x-rays (Bell and Loop, 1971), electronic fetal monitoring (Banta and Thacker, 1976b), Cesarean sections (Marieskind, 1979), and clinical laboratory testing (Schroeder and Showstack, 1979). In particular, so-called "defensive medicine" seems to encourage the excessive use of diagnostic tests.

Malpractice may be linked to technology in another way. The overemphasis on technology and diminishment of the caring function of medicine can lead to dehumanization of the doctor–patient relationship. Some observers relate the incidence of malpractice litigation to a deterioration of this relationship (Jonas, 1977; Department of Health, Education, and Welfare, 1973).

Almost all malpractice claims follow injury of the patient, including failure to recover (Department of Health, Education, and Welfare, 1973). An important problem is that it is often not possible to determine the cause of medical outcomes, including medical injuries. In this situation, the legal standard for practice used is often the most frequent pattern of use. Several recent developments have the potential to create a more appropriate standard. The Consensus Development Conferences sponsored by the National Institutes of Health synthesize information about existing technologies. Such evaluations also form part of the mandated responsibility of the National Center for Health Care Technology. Information from evaluations, rather than existing patterns of use, could become standards of appropriate care. The Professional Standards Review Organizations (PSROs) and other private activities to review quality of care could apply any guidelines formulated, and providers and courts could refer to them.

Industry Promotion of Its Products

Industry spends a great deal of money and effort promoting its products. This is particularly true of the drug industry, which spends more than one billion dollars a year to convince physicians to use its products. In 1971 the prescription drug industry in the United States spent an approximate $700 million on detail men and women, including samples; $167 million for professional journal and direct mail advertising; $150 million for direct and indirect forms of promotion, such as films, plant tours, convention displays, and so forth; and $3 million for institutional promotion. This expenditure approximated the amount the industry invested in research in that year (Silverman and Lee, 1974, pp. 54–55). In 1978 drug companies spent about $3500 per physician promoting their products (Schifrin, 1980).

As noted, the greatest share of the funds is used for the operations of an estimated 25,000 drug detail men and women who visit physicians, pharmacists, and hospital purchasing agents. While the industry defends this practice as educational, it is clear that the major goal of detail men is to encourage use, not to improve prescribing. Since physicians do not have the time to adequately keep up with the professional literature and lack the training to critically examine it, these detailers have inordinate influence on prescribing habits (Silverman and Lee, 1974, p. 50). When physicians were asked to list the most important sources for information on new drugs, 68 percent specified detail men and women (Dowling, 1970, p. 274).

Although the equivalent system for medical devices has not been well described, it certainly exists. The June 1, 1979 issue of *Hospitals* magazine, which focused on issues concerning medical technology, contained advertisements for neonatal intensive care modules, a linear accelerator, a coronary monitor, and an ECG machine. It also had an advertisement from a maker of CT scanners for material explaining certificate-of-need, and offered information on the firm's scanners. We have been told by hospital administrators that equipment-manufacturer representatives are as pervasive as drug detailers. Device manufacturers also produce promotional materials, including well-done movies with an objective veneer, purporting to show why good patient care requires a new machine.

Many physicians have financial interests in this industry and some promote certain products without identifying their conflict of interest. For example, financial arrangements between physicians and independent clinical laboratories are common (Senate, 1977). Dowling (1970, p. 228) notes that experts in a field are often retained, for a fee, as consultants to the industry and may own stock in the company. In the field of devices, one of the inventors of the electronic fetal monitor helped start a company to make the monitor and profited from its sales while he continued to speak and write scientifically about the value of electronic monitoring (Randal, 1978).

The health care industries have well-organized trade associations which lobby on their behalf. The Pharmaceutical Manufacturers Association has been well established for some time. For medical devices, the Health Industry Manufacturers Association, the National Electrical Manufacturers Association, and the Scientific Apparatus Manufacturers Association have all become visible in Washington in the past several years.

Organization of Medical Care

The growth and complexity of knowledge and technology have stimulated a growing institutionalization of medical practice. In part, this is related to specialization and, in part, is due to the expense and difficulty of providing modern technological services.

Both medical care literature and health policy have underemphasized the importance of the organizational structure of medical care. This is unfortunate, since changes in the rational use of technology will take place in an organizational context.

Technology and the Hospital

The hospital is the most important societal institution involved with medical technology. It is the center for the expanding technology of medicine and it services the sickest people. Medical and surgical specialists tend to orient their practice toward hospital services and procedures.

In 1977, there were 7099 hospitals in the United States, with more than 1.4 million beds. About 5900 of these were short-term general community hospitals, where medical technology is concentrated (American Hospital Association, 1978a).

The main decisionmaker in hospitals is the physician. "The link between the characteristics of potential patients and the cases actually admitted to a hospital is usually indirect. Physicians act as intermediaries, translating the patient's demand for medical care into a demand for the services of particular hospitals. . . ." (Russell, 1979, p. 17). Literature on the adoption of medical technology by hospitals and physicians has been reviewed in Chapter 4. Little work has been done on the implications of hospital structure or size on technology *use* compared with technology *adoption*. Nonetheless, it is intuitively logical that the structure of the hospital also influences use of technology. For example, research has shown that the greater the participation of the hospital administrator and the chief of staff in medical decisions, the lower the cost per case (Shortell et al., 1976).

The place of the hospital in the broader system may also influence technology use. There is a trend in the health care system toward vertical integration (different levels of care in one institution). Some implications of this trend were described in Chapter 4. A more vertically integrated practice could lower overall costs of care as it incorporates a wider range of costs. On the other hand, the greater accessibility of technologies such as diagnostic tests could lead to higher rates of use (Willems, 1979b).

Technology and the Organization of Medical Practice

Although the traditional pattern of medical practice in the United States is solo practice, there is an increasing trend toward groups. Alternatives to the traditionally separate physicians' offices and part-time physician staff for hospitals have developed. Some data have been developed to show how use in such settings may differ from that in the traditional setting.

Most of the literature relating organizational structure to use of technology relates to Health Maintenance Organizations (HMOs), including prepaid groups. Studies of HMOs have focused on their capitation[1] payment method as an important difference from the usual fee-for-service mode. This factor will be discussed in the section on payment. However, prepaid group practices differ in organizational variables and scale as well. All of these factors, as well as their more comprehensive benefit package, may influence technology use. However, studies of different delivery systems have not considered these influential variables separately. Most research on technology use comparing solo and group practice, for example, refers to capitation groups and fee-for-service solo practice, so that the effects of the payment mechanism and the organization are combined.

The differences between solo practice and group practice can be profound. In contrast to the usually fragmented practice setting, an ambulatory group practice can contain several specialties and basic diagnostic facilities. A hospital-based group has its own hospital. A community health center may have dental and social services. There is an attempt by the system to address a wide range of its patients' problems.

In studies of Medicare beneficiaries in HMOs, expenditures were found to be lowest in groups that owned or controlled hospitals (Corbin and Krute, 1975; Weil, 1976). Medicaid beneficiaries in hospital-based and ambulatory groups had lower hospitalization rates than did controls (Gaus

---

[1]Capitation is a method of paying for health services in which the provider receives a set, per capita amount of payment for each person to be covered, regardless of the actual amount of services provided.

et al., 1976). On the other hand, one study reported that the use of laboratory and radiological procedures was higher in an ambulatory capitation group than in solo fee-for-service practices (Hastings et al., 1973). Another study found radiological use lower in a hospital-based capitation group compared to solo fee-for-service practices, but laboratory use higher (Diehr et al., 1978; Richardson et al., 1977). A number of studies have found hospitalization rates in prepaid group practices to be lower than those in the population as a whole (Luft, 1978; Perrott, 1971).

Members of HMOs have been found to experience lower rates of surgery (Donabedian, 1965; Reidel et al., 1975). Tonsillectomy rates have been uniformly lower in HMOs. With that exception, Luft (1978) found no confirmation that HMOs consistently reduce discretionary surgery. It is possible, however, that the diagnostic categories were too broad to detect real differences.

Since more integrated practices are usually larger, they might be able to realize lower costs by taking advantage of economies of scale in the use of skilled personnel and expensive equipment (Reinhardt, 1972; Fein, 1967). Studies of fee-for-service solo and ambulatory group practices have reported some economies of scale in smaller groups, but not in large ones (Evans et al., 1973; Kimbell and Lorant, 1977).

Thus, the literature does not show clearly what the effect of organization of medical practice is on the use of technology. Clearly, prepaid group practices use fewer hospital beds, even after correcting for age, socioeconomic status, and so forth. Otherwise, the literature is scanty and somewhat contradictory. This will be discussed further in the section on payment mechanisms.

Bureaucratization, Physicians, and Technology

As medical practice becomes increasingly institutionalized, it becomes correspondingly bureaucratized. The medical administrator makes more and more of the important decisions in health care, and lay boards may have important influences over technology acquisition or use. National policy is now to promote HMOs, which are complex organizations, partially as a method of rationalizing technology use.

Scientific management and bureaucratic functioning, as exemplified by administrators, are in considerable conflict with professional norms as applied by physicians (Kaluzny, 1974). The bureaucratic model sees health care as an economic good that should be provided in an economically efficient manner, instead of as a service that should be provided by a professional group committed to high quality and ethical practice. The bureaucratic organization calls for a hierarchy of authority, while professional norms call for authority based on expertise. The bureaucracy functions largely by formal rules, while the professional prefers a high degree of discretion and informality (Smith and Kaluzny, 1975, pp. 149–152). The purpose here is not to analyze which value system is more effective, but to point out some of the implications of incorporating administrators and physicians in complex organizations.

One important aspect of institutionalization of practice is that it dilutes the physician's commitment to the intersts of the patient. An organization has multiple interests, including some of those noted above. Economic efficiency for the whole system is often not in the individual patient's best interest. The physician in the organization comes under pressure to satisfy organizational needs. One of these needs may be to avoid "unnecessary" services. While this is a worthwhile goal for society, the individual patient may suffer (Mechanic, 1977).

The institutionalization of medicine is also related to the loss of the caring function of medicine. The organization relieves the physician of continuing responsibility for the patient. The patient does not call the physician at night, but calls the clinic. Failures of the organization are harder to attribute. Accountability may be lessened or lost. The pressures for efficiency tend to lead to a system that rewards good management or the ability to cope with a large work load rather than humane and interested medical care. Consumer control has been posited as a counterforce, but its full effects have not been evaluated (Putnam and Banta, 1976).

The bureaucratic organization has great theoretical advantages in an era of limited resources. The physician's commitment to the best interests of the patient may conflict with the rationing and control of the technology of medicine. The experience of prepaid group practices indicates that control over technology may be more effectively done through such an organization. But an important reason that such control is possible is that the physician's reference group shifts from patients to peers and is influenced by administrators in the organized setting (Friedson, 1961). Thus, the promotion of solutions to overuse of technology through organization may lead to increasing dehumanization of health care. Since that dehumanization is one of the key factors that caused medical technology to become a policy issue, that would indeed be an ironic outcome.

We do not believe that it is inevitable that organizations become impersonal and inhumane. Health policymakers should be cautious in implementing organizational strategies, however, to be sure that they do not discard the best of medical care in the process.

Payment for Medical Services

Payment Methods

The common methods of paying providers for services facilitate, if not encourage, the use of additional services because medical care providers can increase their revenues by providing more services. As discussed in subsequent chapters, higher levels of use fostered by such payment may not be beneficial and safe for the patient, and may not be cost-effective for the society.

Payment methods also affect the distribution of services among different types of technologies. Existing relative fee scales reward more lucratively the physician's time spent using sophisticated technology than they do the time spent taking a patient's history, conducting a physical examination, or counseling a patient (Schroeder and Showstack, 1978). Although the use of sophisticated technology may make a physician more productive in terms of patients or services processed in a given time, that use may well be inappropriate from either the patient's or the system's perspective.

Hospital charge structures and costing procedures also subsidize the expense of some technologies with revenues from others. For example, the unit price for a radiological service may exceed unit costs and generate substantial "profits" for the provider. Such was the situation early in the diffusion of CT scanners (OTA, 1978b). A hospital may use these profits to subsidize other, less prestigious, services, such as the outpatient department. The overall social effect of this "cross-subsidization" is not clear. The price structure encourages the overuse of some technologies, such as radiology, given in the example. But units such as the outpatient department often provide access to medical care for the poor. Changes in the pricing structure, then, have implications for socially desirable ends such as providing medical care to the poor.

Because incentives to provide inappropriate, technology-based services are inherent in present payment methods, alternative methods of payment have been proposed. The major alternative proposed in the United States is prospective reimbursement (Wagner, 1978). With prospective reimbursement, rates of payment are set in advance of the time period in which they will apply. Theoretically, prospective reimbursement places more risk with the providers, who cannot increase rates of payment during that time period.

Depending on the specific form, however, a prospective reimbursement method may have drawbacks similar to present methods. The unit of payment (whether the service, case, person, department, or organization) and methods of determining rates and treating surpluses and deficits have implications for provider behavior. Unless revenue is fixed during a time period, a provider will have little need to choose among alternative technologies.

If revenue is limited and choice among technologies is necessary, physicians might reduce or forgo the use of technologies that have low marginal efficacy, that duplicate others, or that have less costly alternatives. However, other considerations besides payment method promote technology use. The nature of medical training, increasing specialization of physicians, apprehension about malpractice, the national fascination with technology, and present forms of third-party coverage predispose physicians and hospitals to opt for expensive, prestigious technologies.

Lower utilization rates have resulted under systems using a capitation payment to physicians. Since payment is independent of the use of services, subject to specific benefit coverage, physicians face fixed revenue per person, and can increase their revenue by adding enrollees, rather than by increasing technology use. However, capitation payment gives physicians an incentive to skimp on services, because use increases expenses but not revenue. Compared to fee-for-service payment, lower use has occurred under capitation payment for hospital use (Roemer and Shonick, 1973) and for physician services and prescriptions (Alexander, 1967). As discussed above, msot studies of fee-for-service and capitation payment compared solo and group practices, and thus did not consider integration level and benefit coverage, which could also have produced the results noted.

The effect on technology use of prospective reimbursement to hospitals has been conflicting (Applied Management Sciences, 1978; Dowling et al., 1976), perhaps a reflection of the different forms of prospective reimbursement. The few studies also relate to heterogeneous categories of technologies, such as laboratory tests or x-rays, which may mask meaningful differences in the use of more specific technologies.

Besides prospective reimbursement arrangements, other proposals to improve current payment methods suggest using the vehicle of fee schedules. Although continuing specific services as the units of payment, such lists of rates would be developed in advance of the applicable time period. Hadley and his colleagues (1979) support such an approach in the context of contending that physicians create demand for their own services, but this ability has limits. They cite evidence from the Economic Stabilization Program in the United States and national health insurance in Canada that physicians respond to changes in relative fees and to controls on fees. The policy implication is to construct fee schedules to produce desirable variations among technologies, specialities, and geographical areas. Their evidence also suggests, however, that use and total expenditures increase when limits are placed on fees and justifies investigation into the types of technologies that are affected and whether or not the benefits are worth the costs. One possibility discussed is to tie annual fee increases to experienced and desired growth in physicians' income, as some Canadian provinces have done.

Third-Party Coverage

A consensus exists that third-party coverage of medical care has increased use of and expenditures on medical technology (Feldstein and Taylor, 1977; Russell, 1979). Whereas having to pay for a service ordinarily restrains use of that service, third-party payment for medical technologies lessens or removes the financial considerations. At the time of service, patients bear less cost, and employers or government may share the premium expense. Physicians and hospitals face less risk of bad debts and exercise less restraint from consideration of their patients' finances (Evans, 1974).

One would expect the extent of coverage to affect the use of technologies, as it has their adoption. As described in Chapter 4, coverage of inpatient services has been fairly complete, but coverage of preventive and rehabilitative technologies has been spotty. As the percentage of hospital revenues accounted for by health insurance grew from 60 percent in 1950, to 90 percent in 1975, the cost of a hospital day rose from $16 to $152 (Congressional Budget Office, 1977).

Data on the use of specific technologies are generally lacking. It seems clear that once adopted, many hospital technologies are underutilized (Cromwell et al., 1975). For those with high fixed costs, such as x-ray units, the implication is higher per unit costs than if fewer units each performed more examinations.

The spectacular rise in the use of ancillary services provided by hospital-based physicians, such as radiologists and pathologists, is related to specialization and payment method as well as third-party coverage. From 1968 to 1971, more intense use of nine such medical services accounted for about 40 percent of the increase in hospital operating costs (Redisch, 1974). These hospital-based physicians receive higher incomes from greater volume of services, but their incomes are usually unrelated to the expenses of providing those services. The hospital typically provides the facilities and absorbs those expenses. In turn, most hospital payments from third parties are based on reasonable cost incurred, so that higher revenues cover the facilities and their operating costs (Congressional Budget Office, 1977).

With fee-for-service payment methods, expansion of coverage to technologies in ambulatory settings appears to increase overall costs and use (Lewis and Keairnes, 1970; Roemer, 1958). The growth of diagnostic radiological practices and surgical centers may be the result of expanded coverage to these settings. Whether these facilities have added to total use and expenditures and whether the benefits are worth the cost have not been analyzed (Willems, 1976b).

The case of renal dialysis is a striking example of the effect of third-party coverage on use. In 1972, when legislation extended Medicare coverage to patients with end-stage renal disease, about 5000 people were on dialysis, 40 percent of them in home programs. By 1976 more than 17,000 patients were on dialysis, but only 24 percent in home programs (Rettig, 1979c). Home dialysis is much less expensive that dialysis in other sites: about $7000 for home dialysis, $17,000 for limited care dialysis, and $25,000 for in-hospital dialysis, in 1972 (Rettig, 1979a). With Medicare coverage, more severely ill patients who required hospital care entered dialysis. But the specifics of Medicare coverage discouraged the use of home dialysis. Patients on home dialysis personally had to bear much higher costs, and providers had little incentive to assume the burden of training and managing home patients. Recent legislation has increased coverage of expenses connected with home dialysis and has provided financial incentives for providers to supervise home patients (Rettig, 1979a).

Empirical studies have shown that coverage for preventive services appears to have little effect on patients' use of them (Lairson and Swint, 1978). The exception, however, is use by the poor, who have higher rates with greater coverage (Colle and Grossman, 1978; Cauffman et al., 1967). This finding has implications for Medicare, whose statute prohibits payment for most immunizations and other preventive services, such as examinations for eyeglasses and hearing aids. Since many of the elderly are in lower income groups, self-payment may deter their use of pneumococcal or influenza vaccine—preventive services specifically recommended for the elderly (Willems, 1979b).

The methods that insurers have used to pay physicians have a built-in inflationary bias for price and expenditures (Showstack et al., 1979). Indemnity companies may use relative value studies to develop fee schedules. With unit fees or prices constant, physicians have been observed to bill for additional services or shift use and billing to more complex, expensive services. Medicare and many Medicaid programs use the "usual, customary, reasonable method" under which physicians receive the lesser of 1) the actual charge, 2) that physician's usual charge, 3) the customary charge in the area, or 4) the reasonable amount justified. Since future levels of payment are based on past charges, physicians have an incentive to bill at a high rate. Since 1975 Medicare has limited annual increases, but the limits are generous: for 1978 they were 42.6 percent above 1971 charge levels (Showstack et al., 1979).

Thus, although the data are not complete, it is clear that insurance coverage has a profound effect on technology use—overall, probably in the direction of increasing it. By the same logic, insurance coverage could be used as a positive planning or resource allocation tool.

Discussion

This chapter has underscored the complexity of the factors influencing use of medical technologies. Despite the limitations of available data on use, it is clear that multiple factors are important. Public policy, in attempting to influence the use of medical technologies, must become more aware of these factors and their ripple effects. Researchers should focus more on the use of technologies and factors promoting or retarding such use. While organizational, legal, and financial factors tend to support the underlying values of society, relatively small changes in such factors could have great implications for promoting rational (or irrational) use of technologies. In an era when public and private policy seems to be turning away from regulatory interventions and seeking to structure incentives to promote desirable social goals, these factors merit particular attention.

6
Evaluation of Efficacy and Safety

> Be not swept off your feet by the vividness of the impression, but say, "Impression, wait for me a little. Let me see what you are and what you represent. Let me try you."
>
> Epictetus

Efficacy and safety are the basic starting points in evaluating the overall utility of a medical technology. If a technology is not efficacious, it should not be used, and if its efficacy is unknown, statements about its overall value cannot be made. For example, ethical issues would not have been raised regarding amniocentesis if it had been demonstrated to be lacking in benefit or clearly unsafe. In addition, efficacy and safety data are needed to evaluate the cost effectiveness of a technology (see Chapter 7). Neither the need for a technology nor its appropriate use in medical care can be established without reliable and valid information on efficacy and safety. Federal programs to regulate and to provide medical care and medical technology depend on efficacy and safety information to assure wise decisions.

Information obtained from assessments of the efficacy and safety of new and existing medical technologies might help ensure that technologies demonstrated to have potential benefits with acceptable risks are made available rapidly, might constrain the diffusion and use of technologies which either lack efficacy or cause excessive harm, and might guide appropriate use of all technologies.

The Federal Government is concerned with questions of efficacy and safety because of its general role as protector of the public and its specific role as developer and user of medical technology. Because public funds pay about 40 percent of national health expenditures (National Center for

---

This chapter is based on *Assessing the Efficacy and Safety of Medical Technologies* by the Office of Technology Assessment, and much of the material is excerpted from that report.

Health Statistics, 1980, p. 237), concerns have naturally arisen about the benefits of medical care. Such questions seem certain to lead to increasing scrutiny of medical care expenditures and accelerated efforts to generate information regarding the benefits derived from the use of medical technologies. Indeed, a variety of Federal programs are hampered in carrying out their mandated tasks by lack of such information.

The concepts of efficacy and safety have not been suddenly discovered or created. They have always existed in medical thought. In an intuitive sense, an efficacious and safe medical technology is one that "works" and causes no undue harm. That statement may sound naive to individuals working in the field of health today. However, for a major portion of the history of medicine, efficacy and safety were measured by that intuitive standard. It still lies at the heart of medical practice, but the meaning and measurement of those concepts have evolved with increased sophistication of scientific methods in medicine.

Efficacy

There is no shortage of definitions for efficacy (Table 6–1); nor is there a lack of confusion relating to distinctions between terms such as efficacy, effectiveness, benefit, and efficiency. Despite the sometimes substantial differences among the various interpretations of efficacy, one can isolate four critical factors that, taken together, form a comprehensive view of the concept.

The factors are: Benefit to be achieved, medical problem giving rise to use of the technology, population affected, and conditions of use under which the technology is applied.

Benefit

The question of what outcomes represent benefits is not simply answered. Outcome criteria have usually been restricted to measurement of mortality and morbidity; less consideration has been given to life expectancy (longevity) or psychosocial and functional factors (Brook, 1974; Brook et al., 1976). The definition of benefit to be used will vary depending on the goals of the investigator and the type of technology being assessed. As our society comes to value psychosocial and functional benefits more, one would expect to see more attempts to measure such outcomes and more use of such studies in developing policy toward specific technologies.

The range of relevant outcomes can be considered in regard to a particular technology (McPeek et al., 1977). For example, the benefit re-

Table 6–1.
Selected Definitions of "Efficacy"

Source	Term defined	Definition	Relation to four factors (See text)
Federal Food, Drug, and Cosmetic Act	Effectiveness, Efficacy (interchangeable)	A drug is effective if it has "the effect it purports or is represented to have under the conditions of use prescribed, recommended, or suggested in the proposed labeling thereof"	Benefit: Explicit Population affected: Implied Medical problem: Explicit Condition of use: Explicit, but incomplete
A. Cochrane in *Effectiveness and Efficiency*	Efficacy (interchangeable with effectiveness)	"The effect of a particular medical action in altering the natural history of a particular disease for the better"	Benefit: Explicit Population affected: Not included Medical problem: Explicit Condition of use: Not included
World Health Organization	Efficacy	Benefit or utility to the individual of the service, treatment regimen, drug, preventive or control measure advocated or applied	Benefit: Explicit Population affected: Explicit Medical problem: Explicit Condition of use: Not included
Discursive Dictionary of Health Care	Efficacy (as a variant of effectiveness)	"The degree to which diagnostic, preventive, therapeutic, or other action or actions (undertaken under ideal circumstances) achieves the desired result"	Benefit: Explicit Population affected: Not included Medical problem: Not included Conditions of use: Explicit
Office of Technology Assessment	Efficacy	The probability of benefit to individuals in a defined population from a medical technology applied for a given medical problem under ideal conditions of use	Benefit: Explicit Population affected: Explicit Medical problem: Explicit Conditions of use: Explicit

Source: Office of Technology Assessment. *Assessing the Efficacy and Safety of Medical Technologies.* Washington, D.C.: U.S. Government Printing Office, 1978.

sulting from use of diagnostic technologies can be examined at five levels (Fineberg et al., 1977a):

1. Technical capability—Does the device perform reliably and deliver accurate information?
2. Diagnostic accuracy—Does use of the device permit accurate diagnoses?
3. Diagnostic impact—Does use of the device replace other diagnostic procedures, including surgical exploration and biopsy?
4. Therapeutic impact—Do results obtained from the device affect planning and delivery of therapy?
5. Patient outcome—Does use of the device contribute to improved health of the patient?

If it is assumed that the function of a diagnostic technology, such as skull x-ray, is to perform accurate diagnoses of individuals' illnesses, the evaluation of benefit concentrates on the second level. If the diagnostic technology is expected to affect therapy or eventual patient outcome, then the fourth and fifth levels would be examined. Studies at the fourth and fifth levels may be difficult to conduct because of such factors as the length of time required for followup studies. As a result of this difficulty and the emphasis on diagnostic accuracy, evaluations in terms of therapeutic planning and patient outcome are infrequently performed (Banta and McNeil, 1978).

The specification of benefit is often difficult for other classes of technologies as well. For example, is the efficacy of coronary bypass surgery to be evaluated in terms of its ability to give relief from symptoms (e.g., pain) or in terms of increased longevity for the patient? Thus, two different measures of benefit may possibly yield two different statements of efficacy for the same technology.

Medical Problem

A technology's efficacy can be evaluated only in relation to the diseases or medical conditions for which it is applied. The specification of medical problems is complex and can lead to controversy regarding the evaluation of the efficacy of a particular technology. For example, hysterectomies have been performed for a variety of medical conditions: premalignant states and localized cancers, descent or prolapse of the uterus, and obstetric catatrophes such as septic abortion. They may also be perfomed as prophylaxis to avoid possible later cancer or pregnancy. If the efficacy of hysterectomy has been estimated for one of these diseases or medical conditions, it cannot be assumed automatically that the procedure will have similar efficacy for the others.

Population Affected

The effect of a medical technology varies, depending on the individual treated. Sometimes, however, enough uniformity of effect exists to permit careful generalizations (Hill, 1952, 1971). These generalizations, or extrapolations, apply to the specific population type within which the original observations were made and should be supported by valid and reliable statistical techniques. For example, in the late 1960s the Veterans Administration (VA) conducted a multi-institutional controlled clinical trial of treatment for hypertension using the drugs hydrochlorothiazide, reserpine, and hydralazine. The treatment was shown to be efficacious for patients with diastolic blood pressure above 105 mm of mercury. However, all the patients in the trial were males. Thus, the treatment could be considered to be efficacious (based on that trial and other evidence) for the population studied—males—but no automatic assumptions can be made concerning its efficacy for females.

Conditions of Use

The outcome of the application of a medical technology is partially determined by the skills, knowledge, and abilities of physicians, nurses, and other health personnel; by the quality of the drugs, equipment, and institutional settings; and by support systems used by those personnel during the application. Cardiac surgery, for example, may result in a better outcome when conducted by skillful, well-trained surgeons who frequently perform such operations than when conducted by surgeons who rarely use that technology. A situation where the physician is skillful and experienced, medication is administered carefully, and the patient receives the best care possible must be described as ideal. By definition, not all physicians are the most skillful, and not all conditions of use are of the highest possible quality. Thus, it is valuable to have an outcome measure that is not dependent on the differing variables inherent in *average* conditions of use. Efficacy is this measure. By defining efficacy as benefit under ideal conditions of use, a reasonably consistent measure for that factor is introduced. No conditions of use are absolutely ideal but, for most purposes, carefully controlled research settings may serve as a substitute for ideal circumstances.

When the four factors described above are specified for the application of a specific medical technology, a comprehensive statement has been made as to that technology's efficacy. These four variables or factors can serve to define the concept of efficacy.

Efficacy: The probability of benefit to individuals in a defined population from a medical technology applied for a given medical problem under ideal conditions of use.

This book differentiates efficacy from effectiveness. Effectiveness is concerned with the benefit of a technology under average conditions of use. Though they can be viewed as distinct, efficacy and effectiveness are closely related concepts. The effectiveness of a technology is estimated by methods similar to those used to estimate its efficacy; however, estimating effectiveness is often more difficult because of the absence of rigorously controlled settings.

Safety

Safety, like efficacy, is a relative concept: no technology is ever completely safe or completely efficacious. In the beginning of this chapter, a safe technology was described intuitively as one that "causes no undue harm." Despite the apparent simplicity of that informal definition, it reflects a critical property of the concept of safety: safety represents a value judgment of the acceptability of risk. Risk can be thought of as a measure of the probability and severity of harm to human health (Lowrence, 1976, p. 94). This definition of risk implies that investigators and policymakers should be concerned with both the nature of the risk and the probability of its occurrence.

Thus, if the risks of using a medical technology are acceptable (to the patient, physician, society, or other appropriate decisionmaker), the technology may be considered "safe" in that instance (Cousins, 1976).

As with efficacy, several factors must be specified when risk and safety are discussed: The *medical problem* for which the technology being evaluated is applied, the *population affected*, and the *conditions of use* under which the technology is applied.

For our purposes, then, risk may be defined as follows:

Risk: The probability of an adverse or untoward outcome's occurring and the severity of the resultant harm to health of individuals in a defined population, associated with use of a medical technology applied for a given medical problem under specified conditions of use.

This definition covers risk under ideal (research) settings, under average or typical settings, and under conditions where quality is below average. This coverage is afforded by the specification of "conditions of use." Normally, when "efficacy and safety" judgments are being discussed, risk is assumed to be measured under ideal conditions of use.

Given this definition of risk, safety can be specified.

Safety: A judgment of the acceptability of risk in a specified situation.

Efficacy and Safety

Efficacy and safety are separate concepts; they can be measured and discussed as distinct properties of a medical technology. Efficacy is defined in terms of a benefit; safety, in terms of a risk. There are, though, many similarities between the two concepts. Neither efficacy nor safety is absolute. Both are discussed in terms of probability and magnitude of benefit or harm. Most important, however, each can be fully evaluated only in terms of the other. A technology may provide benefits, but the value of those benefits depends in part on the risks involved in using the technology. Thus, any use of a medical technology involves a compromise, a trade-off, between potential benefit and risk. It is this type of trade-off that physicians have been analyzing and taking action on throughout the history of medicine.

An example of the need to balance benefit and risk is the epidemic of retrolental fibroplasia (a form of blindness) in babies in the 1930s. Nearly one-fourth of all premature infants weighing less than four pounds at birth were afflicted. Eventually, it was recognized that high levels of oxygen given to premature infants was the cause (Lambert, 1978, pp. 97–101). By 1955 evidence had accumulated that indicated it was possible to keep the oxygen level of the infant's blood normal without causing the disease. There had been no controlled study of oxygen in premature infants until oxygen was suspected as the cause (Silverman, 1977). The case also illustrates that the risk of an intervention often appears only after it has been in use for some time, emphasizing the need for caution in the implementation of technologies and for some method of periodically reexamining experience with technologies in use.

Efficacy and safety are usually represented as statistical concepts. Benefit and risk are spoken of as probabilities in relation to any one individual. However, it should be kept in mind that those statistics and probabilities are population-based. A woman who undergoes a hysterectomy does not avoid a percentage of her early death. She either receives the entire benefit (e.g., prevention of death due to cervical cancer), or she took the risk of major surgery in order to avoid a cancer that never would have occurred. In this latter case, the risk would outweigh the real medical benefit. Psychological benefit and avoidance of other potential conditions, of course, make our characterization of the example simplistic but do not defeat the concept. Another example is provided by electronic fetal monitoring. Some fetuses will benefit; all are put at risk. These benefits and risks do not divide equally. The potential benefit to many fetuses is low or nonexistent, yet they are put at equal risk. The problem is that, even with such considerations, information on efficacy and safety *are* probabilistic. The goal should be to narrow and refine as much as possible the population to which a technology is applied.

Technologies are used within a cultural context, and this context has often overridden considerations of efficacy and safety. Our argument is not that efficacy and safety must take precedence over society's culture-based judgments but, rather, that such subjugation of medical indications should only take place in the presence of full information that it is being done. Normally, it should take a profound cultural imperative to override considerations of efficacy and safety. This has not always been the case. The point may be illustrated by the use in the 1800s and early 1900s of clitoridectomy (surgical removal of the clitoris), female circumcision, and oophorectomy (surgical removal of the ovaries) for the treatment of psychological disorders. Use of these procedures was based on an image of women largely rejected today. Since women were considered responsible for bringing up children, it was thought that overloading their nervous systems would have deleterious effects on their offspring. Thus, these surgical procedures were used as late as 1946 to check female masturbation, which physicians felt would arouse women's naturally boundless but usually repressed sexual appetites and lead to mental disorders. Although these procedures are now abandoned, at least for that indication, female surgery of uncertain benefit still goes on. For example, the rates of hysterectomy and breast surgery in this country are more than double those in England and Wales (Bunker, 1970). It does not seem farfetched to suggest that historical and cultural attitudes toward women are related to this medical situation (Barker-Benfield, 1976, pp. 120–121).

Uses and Users of Efficacy and Safety Data

Any person or institution using or directly affecting the use of medical technologies is a user of efficacy and safety information. Patients or consumers of medical care are very important users; yet a great many consumers do not view themselves in this light. They take a relatively passive role in regard to efficacy and safety information. This state of affairs is changing somewhat, with numerous consumer groups taking an active interest in the state of evidence on efficacy and safety (Boston Women's Health Book Collective, 1976). Many Government and private sector programs—for example, several of the grant programs of the Department of Health and Human Services' Health Services Administration (HSA)—also are users of efficacy and safety data who have not seen themselves as being directly concerned with such information. HSA, for example, may award a grant to a community for the establishment of certain specific health services. The agency does not require that technological services provided with these funds be of demonstrated efficacy and safety. This situation represents a passive or indirect use of efficacy and safety information because the usefulness of the grant program depends in part on the effectiveness, and thus the efficacy, of the service purchased. Direct and active users of efficacy and safety information include physicians, biomedical and health services researchers, nurses, other health professionals, many public and private third-party payers, government regulatory programs, medical schools, and so on. Table 6–2 lists many of the users and their sources of information.

Estimating Efficacy and Safety

Techniques used for estimating efficacy and safety range from the informal methods of individual physicians to randomized clinical trials with complex methodological designs. No technique is universally applicable for every medical technology. In many instances less complex methods may be more appropriate than the more sophisticated approaches. Frequently, combinations of techniques are used. This section describes five techniques used in evaluating safety and efficacy: preclinical, informal, epidemiological and statistical, controlled clinical trials, and formal synthesis.

Preclinical

Many medical technologies are evaluated in biochemical and animal tests prior to human experimentation. These preclinical tests may be part of the developmental effort, or a requirement for Federal or private approval, or both. The required tests may be of two types: 1) preliminary evidence to gain the right to test with humans and 2) performance standard compliance to establish marketability.

Table 6–2.
Users of Efficacy and Safety Information

User	Action Taken on the Basis of Efficacy and Safety Information	Major Sources of Information
Non-Federal, private:		
Physicians (and nurses, other health professionals)	Clinical decisionmaking relative to diagnosis, treatment, and prevention of health problems Decisions to adopt new technologies Publishing, communicating to professional associations, colleagues, etc.	Own experience Colleagues Professional meetings Professional literature Detail men, other manufacturers' representatives
Professional associations	Set standards for use of technologies Assess competence for certification, etc. Communication to membership, etc.	Professional literature Experience of members and other health professionals
Schools of medicine or public health	Instruction Set agendas for future research	Knowledge and experience of faculties Professional literature
Private sector third-party payers	Decisions to place a technology on the coverage schedule Decisions to reimburse for specific uses of a technology	Professional opinion Professional literature Associations
Federal Government programs:		
Food and Drug Administration (PHS)	Decisions to allow investigational use of drugs or devices Decisions to allow marketing of drugs or devices Decisions to allow products to stay on market	Manufacturer or sponsor Professional literature Staff knowledge Outside professional advisors

Medicare program (HCFA)	See private third-party payers	National Center for Health Care Technology (PHS) NIH, and other Federal programs See private third-party payers
Medicaid program (HCFA)	See private third-party payers (HCFA recommends such decisions but the states have the decision authority)	Medicare decisions See private third-party payers
National Institutes of Health (PHS)	Decisions on research agendas Decisions on demonstration and control programs Dissemination of information	Research conducted at or supported by NIH Professional literature Outside advisors Staff knowledge
Health Resources Administration (PHS)	Set national guidelines for health planning Develop planning guidance for certificate-of-need determinations	Other Federal agencies Contracts with private organizations Professional literature
Office of Professional Standards Review Organizations (HCFA)	Set guidelines for medical care reviews Set guidelines for reviews of institutional admissions and length-of-stay	See Health Resources Administration

Source: Office of Technology Assessment. *Assessing the Efficacy and Safety of Medical Technologies.* Washington, D.C.: U.S. Government Printing Office, 1978.

Animal testing provides a guide to potential therapeutic activity as well as capacity to induce toxicity (Cooper, 1971; 1972). Determining the degree of toxicity, or safety, is the major function of animal studies. The accuracy of animal models in determining the probable effects of drugs on people is a controversial issue. Despite some of the inherent problems in utilizing animals, they are acceptable models for cancer studies and probably should be regarded as reasonable precursors to clinical studies (OTA, 1977, p. 5).

Informal

Despite the increasing need to formally estimate the efficacy and safety of medical technologies, most evaluation is informal (White, 1968; OTA, 1978a, p. 94).

Personal experience, dominated by qualitative impressions, is perhaps the oldest and most common informal method of judging the efficacy and safety of a medical technology. The control groups, if any, are often hypothetical and are primarily envisioned as experiencing the end result that would occur if there were no clinical intervention (Cooper). However, personal knowledge of the patient may promote beneficial adjustments to the type and level of treatment. Perhaps more important, personal experience is the primary method that determines whether or not a medical technology is adopted into widespread practice (Coleman et al., 1966; Kaluzny, 1974).

Peer experience is more explicit than personal experience; information may be exchanged by personal communication, journal articles, pamphlets, and the like. There is limited control over the scientific quality of these technical assessments. Peer interaction is, however, the core concept of professional consensus activities.

Professional consensus represents a method of systematically tapping the often extremely valuable opinions and experience of practicing physicians and medical researchers.

Professional consensus can arise either informally and spontaneously or in a more structured fashion. Informal consensus is reflected in a common perception among practitioners of the appropriate use of a technology. It will often be based on the factors mentioned above—personal experience and peer interaction—and spread through informal contacts, professional meetings, and journal articles. A more structural approach to professional consensus development occurs when expert practitioners and researchers are brought together to share their opinions as to the benefits and risks of a particular technology. Professional societies have often been the agent of this type of activity. The "technical consensus-building" efforts of the National Institutes of Health (to be described later) draw upon the experience and opinion of practitioners, and the result is often a consensus similar to that produced by the professional societies. At times, however, the NIH activities are more formalized and are based heavily on more formal methods of evaluation, such as controlled clinical trials, and possess many of the characteristics of the formal synthesis technique, described below.

It is important to point out that many medical advancements have properly and successfully proceeded without rigorous statistical methodology of evaluation. For example, vitamin B12 treatment for pernicious anemia clearly is justified.

Epidemiology

Epidemiology is the study of the determinants and the distribution of diseases and injuries in human populations. The methods of epidemiology are often used to study the impact of medical interventions. They may be classified as follows (MacMahon et al., 1960, p. 32):

1. Descriptive epidemiology: Description of the distribution of disease, comparing its frequency in different populations and in subgroups of the population.
2. Formulation of hypotheses: Hypotheses are developed that are designed to explain the observed distribution of disease.
3. Analytic epidemiology: Observational studies designed to examine the hypotheses directly.
4. Experimental epidemiology: Experimental studies in human populations. The major type of study used in evaluating technology is the controlled clinical trial. Because of its importance and prevalent use, it will be described below in a separate section.

Sometimes these methods proceed as listed. However, because of contributions to knowledge made by other disciplines such as clinical medicine and biomedical research (see Chapter 3), any, none, or all of these methods may be used in investigations of disease and its treatment.

Descriptive studies have often established links between interventions and outcomes. The classic epidemiological investigation was that of Snow in 1855, in which he established that contaminated drinking water was responsible for an outbreak of cholera. Removal of the handle from the pump of the offending water supply ended the outbreak (MacMahon et al., 1960, p. 33).

Investigation of the association between the regular use of drinking water with greater than average concentrations of fluoride and low rates of dental caries led to experiments with fluoridation of drinking water of selected populations (MacMahon et al., 1960, p. 33). However, descriptive epidemiology is probably more important in determining safety. Even descriptive marketing and manufacturing data may provide critical information on safety—for example, partly through such data, atomizers containing isoproterenol were linked to unexpected deaths with cardiac arrhythmia. Although these studies have inherent problems, they have the advantage of utility, low cost, and quick results (Colombo, 1977; Mausner and Bahn, 1974).

Analytic studies may be done retrospectively, if existing data are adequate, or prospectively. Collecting data prospectively has the major disadvantage of being laborious, time-consuming, and expensive. An interesting, and very expensive, analytic study was conducted on the population of Framingham, Massachusetts. That study followed more than 4000 people for a number of years, and the data gathered on risk factors for heart disease led to a large controlled clinical trial to determine the effectiveness of different methods of convincing people to modify their behavior as an approach to preventing deaths from coronary disease (MacMahon et al., 1960, p. 212).

Epidemiological and statistical methods are now used frequently in computer modelling and multiple regression techniques to examine the efficacy of medical interventions; for example, obstetric technologies (Neutra et al., 1978; Williams and Hawes, 1979).

Controlled Clinical Trials

All subjects who agree to participate in controlled clinical trials are normally assigned to experimental and control groups; they are assigned to either of these groups randomly. In a controlled clinical trial intended to assess efficacy and safety, the experimental group would be treated or diagnosed by the technology under examination; usually the control group would be either treated by an established standard technology or given a placebo. However, in some cases, a standard technology is administered to one of the study groups, while a second (control) group receives no treatment.

Many controlled clinical trials require a long period of time and large commitments of money, resources, and subjects. The National Institutes of Health (NIH) estimated that the total amount of money[1] expended for trials

---

[1] The total amount here refers to the entire cost of completing trials that were underway in FY 1975.

underway in fiscal year 1975 (new starts and continuing studies) was $641.8 million for 755 trials.[2]

Randomized controlled trials are the most useful when: (1) the benefit of a new technology is uncertain, and (2) the relative benefits of existing therapies are disputed (Byar et al., 1976). There is much statistical theory that supports the scientific utility of such randomization procedures in clinical trials. Byar et al. discussed three major advantages to randomization. First, and most familiar, bias may be eliminated from the assignment of treatment. Secondly, randomization prevents bias with respect to variables that exist in the experiment but are not directly considered in the design. This allows comparison between treatment groups. The third advantage of randomization is the validity of the statistical tests of significance that are used to compare treatments. It should be noted that complete randomization may be inappropriate under certain circumstances; in such cases modifications in the randomizing process may be used (Greenberg, 1959).

There are many areas of controversy surrounding the use of randomized clinical trials, perhaps the greatest of which is ethical. Arguments against randomization and other aspects of these trials are based on a concern for both patient and physician rights and responsibilities. The section "Social Values and the Evaluation of Medical Technologies," in Chapter 8, discusses this issue more fully.

Formal Synthesis

The assessment of a specific medical technology may include one or more studies that use any or all of the techniques previously described. If the evidence clearly supports or rejects the relative utility of a treatment, then the analysis of efficacy and safety may be complete (though it may need periodic reexamination). In many cases, however, the evidence does not lead to such an unequivocal decision. Consequently, the technique of synthesis may be used both to evaluate all pertinent information, which may range from informal to detailed statistical studies, and to convey its findings to the medical community.

Synthesis involves a "putting together" of all available information. It is more than a summary of opinion and research findings. What is synthesized is not simply the conclusions or findings of existing studies and other information sources but, rather, the results of critical analyses (methodological and policy-related) of those conclusions and findings and of the "current wisdom." It is really a process of analysis-synthesis-analysis-judgment. Exist-

[2] Trials supported by the NIH vary widely in costs. One of the most expensive, the Multiple Risk Factor Intervention Trials (MRFIT), is budgeted at $115.7 million.

ing information is analyzed; the results of these analyses are merged and then analyzed for what can be formally stated and, often, recommended about the benefits, risks, and indications for appropriate use of the technology in question. Through this process of tearing down existing information and blending it to form decision-relevant statements, new information is in effect created. The process depends on a close cooperation of those with data on the effects of technology and those with a sensitivity to the information needs of practitioners, bureaucrats, and other decisionmakers.

Current Assessment Activities

National Center for Health Care Technology

The National Center for Health Care Technology (NCHCT) is the newest Federal agency concerned directly with evaluation of medical technologies, and it is the first designed to address concerns about technology in a comprehensive and systematic fashion.

The Center was created by Public Law 95-623 in November of 1978. It and two other centers (the National Center for Health Statistics and the National Center for Health Services Research) are organizationally located under a single Deputy Assistant Secretary, for purposes of coordination and cooperation (see organizational chart of HHS in Appendix B).

The NCHCT is to "set priorities for technology assessment, and encourage, conduct, and support assessments, research, demonstrations, and evaluations concerning health care technology" (Office of the Assistant Secretary for Health). Although its mandate includes different types of assessments of technologies—including efficacy, safety, economic, social, and ethical issues—one of the most significant roles it plays is related to efficacy and safety information. That is, the NCHCT is to provide recommendations to the Medicare program of the Health Care Financing Administration (HCFA) on whether to include specific technologies in the reimbursement schedule. Interestingly, the intent of the Center is to provide HCFA with information on costs as well as efficacy and safety, although current interpretation of the Medicare laws does not include costs as a criteria for allowing reimbursement for a particular technology.

The establishment of this Center would seem to provide a badly needed focus for the diverse and uncoordinated activities of HHS in regard to medical technology (OTA, 1978a; Health Technology Management, 1977). It does have the potential to serve as this focus. However, it is a staff office, not an operating (line) agency and, so far, has only limited staff and funds. More important, the Center will depend on the good will and personal authority of HHS administrators for its success: it has extremely limited organizational authority to compel cooperation between relevant agencies. One way that NCHCT *is* linked with other agencies is through its National Council on Health Care Technology. In addition to the public members of the council, there are a large number of ex officio members representing such organizations as HCFA, NIH, FDA, CDC, the VA, the PSRO program, and the National Council on Health Planning. Other efforts to establish linkage are planned cooperative and joint studies with HCFA and NIH, among others. Despite some potential weaknesses, the NCHCT is an important recognition of the necessity for approaching medical technologies as a generic class of technologies giving rise to effects that need to be carefully and comprehensively assessed and managed.

Food and Drug Administration

The Food and Drug Administration (FDA) of the Department of Health and Human Services is one of the principal Federal regulatory agencies designed to protect the health of the American public. FDA regulates the transfer of certain medical technologies from the level of medical researcher to the level of health practitioner and consumer. The agency particularly emphasizes regulation in those areas where consumers cannot make reasonably informed judgments.

PRESCRIPTION DRUGS. FDA is responsible for implementing the Food, Drug, and Cosmetic Act of 1938 and its amendments. This Act mandates Federal regulation of all drugs. As the Act's principal enforcer, FDA is required to approve all new drugs before they are marketed. Such approval is contingent upon the demonstrated efficacy and safety of the new drug.

The requirement that the efficacy of a new drug be demonstrated before approval was added to the Act by amendment in 1962. Previously, the 1938 Act restricted FDA's review to the safety of drugs. Therefore, the fact that a particular drug was not shown to be efficacious could not, in most cases, serve as the basis for disapproval of its marketing application.

Two statements from the 1962 amendments form the basis for FDA's definition of efficacy. The statute requires the FDA Commissioner to refuse approval of a drug marketing application if "there is lack of substantial evidence that the drug will have the effect it purports or is represented to have under the conditions of use prescribed, recommended, or suggested in the proposed labeling thereof. . . ." Substantial evidence is defined in the Act as: "evidence consisting of adequate and well-controlled investigations, including clinical investigations. . . ."

Safety is assessed as a separate factor from efficacy. FDA must weigh the relative benefits and risks associated with the use of drug, and the drug may enter the market only when the benefits derived from its use clearly outweigh the risks.

FDA processes do protect the public from unsafe or inefficacious drugs, and also serve to develop information that can be used by physicians and others to make better decisions on drug use. The problem is that the regulation increases the time necessary to develop and market a drug. Judging the success of the FDA requires weighing the importance of the hypothetical adverse effects avoided against the hypothetical harm resulting from lack of the drug. This requires a value judgment that is difficult to make.

MEDICAL DEVICES. FDA was first provided authority to regulate medical devices in the Food, Drug, and Cosmetic Act of 1938. This Act extended FDA control over foods and drugs and gave FDA new powers with regard to cosmetics and medical devices. Under the Act, the FDA had to prove that a product was in fact dangerous or fraudulent before any action could be taken to remove the product from the market.

The development and use of medical devices have expanded greatly since the passage of the 1938 Act. As a result of the dynamic growth of the industry, more complex, sophisticated, and technologically challenging products were being developed that had the potential to cause serious patient injury or even death. In response to these dangers, Congress enacted the Medical Device Amendments of 1976, which gave FDA significant new authority to ensure the safety and efficacy of medical devices (Banta et al., 1978). Accordingly, they require evaluations of efficacy and safety to be made "weighing any probable benefit to health from use of the device against any risk of injury or illness from such use." To achieve such evaluations, Congress both expanded FDA's operative definition of medical devices and required classification of all devices into one of three regulatory categories, differentiated according to the extent of control necessary to ensure their efficacy and safety.

FDA designed its system of classification and regulatory controls to prevent unnecessary regulation of device manufacturers, while simultaneously providing maximum protection to consumers. Devices placed in the Class I category are subject only to general controls that include premarket notification, adherence to good manufacturing practices, and recordkeeping requirements. Class II medical devices must meet FDA's performance standards, which may relate to their construction, components, ingredients, and properties, such as diagnostic accuracy. A manufacturer must seek premarket approval of a medical device when general controls would not ensure its safety and efficacy and when there is insufficient information available to develop performance standards. Premarket approval is the overriding regulatory requirement for Class III devices. Devices that are life-sustaining, life-supporting, or implanted into the body usually must be placed in the Class III category.

This program is too new to evaluate but does involve the same difficult judgments necessary in deciding on the value of drug regulation.

National Institutes of Health

The National Institutes of Health (NIH) is the principal biomedical research agency of the Federal Government. It was established just after World War II, both to consolidate the government's medical research activities and to conduct, encourage, and support medical research and development. Its support of biomedical R&D is described in Chapter 3. Research conducted by NIH includes studies of drugs, devices, and medical and surgical procedures. These studies usually are accomplished through grant and contract awards to academic and other research institutions. However, NIH generally does not synthesize the evidence regarding efficacy and safety gained from these studies, nor does it actively disseminate their results.

Specific references to efficacy or effectiveness do not appear in any of the NIH legislative authorities. However, NIH concern regarding the efficacy and safety of medical technologies can be assumed from the general language it uses to describe its mission: 1) advancing knowledge and understanding of the normal and pathological processes of the human body, and 2) developing ways in which the providers of medical care can safely and effectively intervene to prevent, treat, or cure disease and disabilities.

CLINICAL TRIAL SUPPORT. Clinical trials provide the basis for the testing and orderly application of fundamental research knowledge. These trials assist in preventing the premature introduction of new diagnostic and treatment modalities into general practice. Often, such trials are the only methods used for testing and evaluating the safety and efficacy of new diagnostic and treatment developments.

NIH investment in both the support and conduct of clinical trials has increased substantially in recent years. Four out of the eleven institutes[3]

---

[3] The four institutes were the National Cancer Institute; the National Heart, Lung, and Blood Institute; the National Institute of Neurological and Communicative Disorders and Stroke; and the National Eye Institute.

nearly tripled their total obligations for clinical trials between 1971 and 1974. In fiscal year (FY) 1975 alone, NIH provided approximately $110 million to support 775 clinical trials; this figure represents 5 percent of the total NIH budget for FY 1975. Completion of these trials was estimated to cost another $345 million (National Institutes of Health, 1977a). For 1976, NIH spent $147 million on 926 clinical trials.[4]

NIH clinical trial expenditures can be classified by three functions of technology: therapeutics, prophylaxis, or diagnosis. Clinical trials investigating therapeutic technologies were predominant in 1975. Information provided by NIH indicates that a total of 535 trials were conducted to test drugs, either in isolation or in combination with another type of technology. Four hundred of these trials tested drugs in isolation. More than 300 trials tested cancer chemotherapies; only 25 evaluated surgical procedures. Eighty-five trials examined diagnostic technologies such as CT scanning for brain tumors and fluorescent scanning in thyroid disease. However, few clinical trials examined the efficacy of screening or early diagnosis. Trials of primary prevention were quite rare.

CONSENSUS DEVELOPMENT. According to NIH, the present process for diffusion of medical technologies "leads to a situation in which the practicing community at large is not prepared to react promptly and in best informed state to rapid advances in technology. . . . While the Food and Drug Administration has stringent requirements for the safety and efficacy of drugs, biologics, and devices, many procedures existing in current medical practice and new interventions entering the medical arena and adopted by practitioners are not amenable to such regulatory action and require more critical appraisal of effectiveness" (National Institutes of Health, 1976). Although there have been many situations in which a clinical trial has firmly established the efficacy and safety of a particular medical technology, there are other situations in which a controlled clinical trial has not been done or in which the results of a clinical trial have been equivocal. Also, in some cases controlled trials may indicate that a technology is of limited benefit. Thus, the technology is efficacious but the value of this limited efficacy must be evaluated by other techniques besides the controlled trials. In some cases clinical trials may be prohibitively expensive. In other cases trials may pose difficult ethical and moral considerations. In such cases clinical experience can be an important factor in determining what use should be made of the technology.

Due to both the inherent limitations in clinical trials and the need for

---

[4] Information on Fiscal Year 1976 clinical trials was provided to OTA by the National Institutes of Health.

improved methods of disseminating research information, NIH initiated a process for developing a consensus among representative experts regarding the proper role of a given medical technology (National Institutes of Health, 1979). NIH calls that process "technical consensus development." Representatives of various segments of the medical community are asked to agree on five issues: the clinical significance of the new findings; the adequacy of efforts to validate efficacy and safety; the need to identify financial, ethical, or other social impacts as points for caution; the need for feasibility demonstrations in community settings; and whether research results are phrased for easy understanding and acceptance by health practitioners (National Institutes of Health, 1977b).

A major example of consensus development application at NIH was the 1977 Meeting on Breast Cancer Screening. The meeting was held to coincide with the completion of a review of the Breast Cancer Detection Demonstration Project (BCDDP), which involved periodic screening of large numbers of women for breast cancer, using clinical history, physical examination, mammography, and thermography. Critics had questioned whether the use of radiation (by mammography) to detect cancers might not subsequently trigger development of malignancies (Bailar, 1977).

NIH convened a 16-member panel composed of scientists, epidemiologists, and physicians from various disciplines, including radiology, medical oncology, surgery, and general medicine. Representatives of the clergy, legal profession, and lay public were also asked to participate on the panel.

After the gathering of evidence, the panel developed 12 recommendations regarding the risks, benefits, and ethical considerations relating to the BCDDP in particular, and screening in general. The recommendations ranged from specific suggestions for determining which risk groups should continue to undergo periodic screening and the appropriate radiation dose, to general recommendations regarding the need for additional research in particular subject areas.

In January 1978, NIH established the position of Associate Director of Medical Applications of Research as a response to the success of the consensus development process. The Associate Director and staff work with individual institutes to increase awareness of each institute's activities in consensus development. Additionally, they coordinate consensus development efforts that involve a number of institutes simultaneously. This office has developed guidelines for methods to be utilized in: 1) the identification of new knowledge pertinent to health care, 2) consensus development conferences, and 3) the dissemination of research information. Planned consensus development conferences for 1980 include CT head and body scanning and cancer screening.

Other Federal Programs

In addition to the three discussed above, many other agencies of the Federal Government play important parts in efficacy and safety assessment. More than a dozen agencies conduct or support biomedical research, some of which involves testing for efficacy and safety. Examples of such agencies are the Veterans Administration and the Department of Defense.

The Alcohol, Drug Abuse, and Mental Health Administration (ADAMHA) is another agency within HHS. It incorporates programs of basic and applied research, service, and training that are relevant to the understanding and treatment of mental illness, drug abuse, and alcoholism, in its three component institutes: the National Institute on Alcohol Abuse and Alcoholism (NIAAA), the National Institute on Drug Abuse (NIDA), and the National Institute of Mental Health (NIMH). Since the 1950s ADAMHA has conducted research to establish the safety and efficacy of medical technologies. In 1975, however, ADAMHA established Treatment Assessment Research (TAR) as a separate research category, specifically designed to study the relative safety and efficacy of various substances and procedures applied to human subjects. This research includes prospective clinical trials, case reports, retrospective surveys, and reanalysis of early data. The three ADAMHA institutes provided $19 million to support TAR in FY 1975.

Other agencies significantly involved in efficacy-related activities are the Health Services Administration, the National Center for Health Services Research, and the Health Standards and Quality Bureau (see discussion of PSROs in Chapter 9).

Private Sector Activities

The private sector supports many activities intended to evaluate the efficacy and safety of medical technologies. In addition, many Federal programs depend upon private sector facilities and personnel to produce much of the data used for evaluations of safety and efficacy. In fact, most federally financed clinical trials take place in private sector hospitals and clinics, many of which are university-affiliated.

The work of individual physicians or medical center research teams has resulted in a number of innovative medical and surgical procedures. Although there are few formal requirements that new procedures be shown to be efficacious before their use, a substantial amount of testing is still conducted with or without Federal funds.

Some professional associations have developed formal mechanisms for reviewing accumulated evidence regarding the proper use of a technology.

In late 1976 the Medical Practice Committee of the American College of Physicians recommended that the College "explore the feasibility of forming an organization to develop a mechanism for the systematic review of the efficacy of diagnostic and therapeutic procedures." The American Academy of Pediatrics has developed recommendations on immunization practices. The American Public Health Association periodically compiles a list of effective preventive and therapeutic procedures for infectious diseases. The Council of Medical Specialty Societies, the American College of Surgeons, and the American College of Physicians have provided advice to the National Blue Shield on the efficacy of lumbodorsal sympathectomy, uterine suspension, and basal metabolic rate determinations—all questionable procedures for which Blue Shield was continuing to reimburse. The American Hospital Association and the American College of Radiology also have been involved in similar activities.

A System for Assessing Efficacy and Safety

The adoption and use of medical technologies by health care professionals should be based on well-validated information regarding their benefits and risks. This statement does not imply that every aspect of every technology must or can be subjected to randomized, controlled clinical trials. It does imply both the existence of accurate and relevant information, which is developed to the extent desired and practical, regarding the effects of technologies and the dissemination of such information to the individuals and groups in need of it.

The model of the process of generating, processing, and disseminating information on efficacy and safety presented below is later compared to the current systems and programs in order to examine whether shortcomings exist in the current systems. The process and related shortcomings are described in terms of efficacy and safety assessment, but much of what is said applies equally well to evaluation of costs, cost effectiveness, and social impacts.

The process may be viewed as an interdependent and nondiscrete flow of four types of actions (see Figure 6–1):

> Identification: Monitoring technologies, selecting those in need of study, and deciding which to study.
> Testing: Conducting the appropriate analyses or trials.
> Synthesis: Collecting and interpreting existing information and the results of the testing step and, usually, making recommendations or judgments of efficacy and safety.

Figure 6–1.
Process for Developing and Disseminating Efficacy and Safety Information.

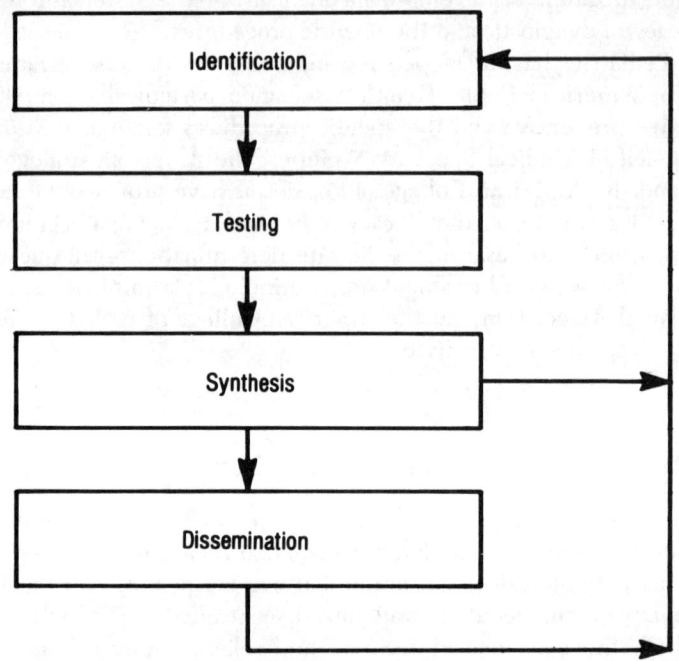

SOURCE: Office of Technology Assessment. *Assessing the Efficacy and Safety of Medical Technologies.* Washington, D.C.: Government Printing Office, 1978.

Dissemination: Providing the synthesized information, or any other relevant information, to the appropriate parties who use or make decisions concerning the use of medical technologies.

Despite the existence of NCHCT, the primary shortcoming in current assessment methods is still the lack of a formal or well-coordinated "system" for developing and disseminating safety and efficacy data. Some elements of the process are operating and performing well. However, the elements are not adequately linked together and do not follow each other logically.

Identification

Presently, there is no complete list or catalogue of either existing medical technologies or those that particularly require assessment for efficacy and safety. Partial lists do exist. The Food and Drug Administration (FDA), for example, has lists of approved drugs and devices. The fact remains, however, that many medical procedures that are not on reimbursement schedules but that are important to assess (bed rest for certain diseases, for example) are not catalogued in one source.

No existing system adequately identifies developing technologies that will need evaluation for safety and efficacy. The National Institutes of Health (NIH) does a yearly study of its clinical trials and publishes a catalogue of those trials it supports. Other agencies, such as the Veterans Administration (VA), have similar catalogues or lists. Through its premarket approval process, FDA gathers information on drugs and devices that are being developed. If medical and surgical procedures were to be evaluated before they came into widespread use, however, some comprehensive system for recognizing them in a timely fashion would be necessary. In addition, FDA and NIH now are required to provide the NCHCT with lists of new and emerging technologies.

Even if funds for, and numbers of, clinical trials were greatly expanded, setting priorities for study would still be necessary, because it is neither possible, nor desirable, to study every efficacy- or safety-related aspect of every medical technology. Several considerations make such sweeping evaluation undesirable. One is the probability of diminishing marginal utility. Presumably, evaluation would reach a point where less and less additional information is gained for the substantial investments of time, money, and other resources that would be required. Another factor is the near impossibility of manipulating and successfully disseminating the tremendous masses of data that would result. Another, and potentially one of the most important issues, is the effect that total assessment might have on incentives for innovation. Even in the current assessment situation some analysts feel that the rate of innovation of medical technology has been lessened. The so-called "drug lag" has been attributed to the Food and Drug Administration (FDA) program regulating safety and efficacy of drugs (Wardell and Lasagna, 1975). However, a careful review article makes it clear that, while FDA definitely increases lag time, it is not possible, based on existing research, to say whether the FDA program is of benefit or harm to the U.S. public in the aggregate (Schifrin and Tayan, 1977). Nonetheless, with increasing regulation of drugs and medical devices, possible harmful feedback effects on innovation and private investment in biomedical R&D must be of concern. Priorities for conducting studies might help to ensure that all areas of medicine, such as prevention, are considered.

Priorities for assessment might include beneficial technologies that are neglected or technologies that are suspected to be useless or dangerous. Technologies that are, or are expected to be, either expensive or widely used also could be given priority. For new technologies, potentially important advances could be assessed rapidly.

One confounding variable in the process of assessment that is especially critical for the identification phase is the stage of development of the technology. Obviously, the farther along the development of a technology is, the better the information about its effects can be. Technologies change as they move from early clinical use, for example, through clinical refinement, to early adoption and their eventual patterns of use in medical practice. Dosages are refined. New generations of devices replace older ones. Surgical techniques are modified. New uses are often added, older ones sometimes abandoned. In other words, the indications for using the technology change, and its potential benefits, risks, and cost change. For example, early in the diffusion of a new technology it may not be desirable to conduct a large-scale randomized controlled clinical trial. At some point, however, as the technology is accepted, such a trial may become highly desirable.

All this implies that criteria for selecting technologies for study need to be sensitive to stage of development as well as being extremely flexible. Trade-offs are inherent. A study done too soon or on a rapidly outdated technology will be of correspondingly limited use; yet delay in assessment could mean that the technology might diffuse before adequate information on its effects was collected. We do not have the answer to this dilemma. We do, however, feel strongly that this aspect of evaluation deserves considerable attention—attention that it is not receiving.

One of the most critical functions of NCHCT is to set these priorities for assessment. That agency has been developing the beginnings of such a process—for example, a priority list has been developed including such technologies as barium enema, ultrasound, and nuclear magnetic resonance—but so far the overall effort has been less than impressive. More attention needs to be placed on the criteria to be used for setting the priorities. Nonetheless, the agency and its advisory council recognize the value of such priority-setting.

In sum, there is little formal process for selecting which technologies are to be studied; indeed, there is not even a widely agreed upon set of priorities for such selection. New drugs and new devices are, however, subject to the FDA market approval process and thus are automatically identified for study, at least in regard to the efficacy and safety claims of the manufacturers.

Testing

The testing phase includes stimulating, requiring, funding, or conducting studies. Shortcomings related to the testing phase center around four issues: (1) the quality of the methodologies for conducting controlled trials, consensus activities, and other tests; (2) the level of financial support, particularly for controlled clinical trials; (3) the relative appropriateness of the questions and technologies being studied; and (4) the number of personnel qualified to conduct such research.

There is no "correct" level of financial support for clinical trials; no one can set an exact figure for the amount that should be invested in trials and other forms of testing. Does the current level of funding, then, represent a shortcoming? This question must be answered affirmatively because important areas of health care are not receiving adequate investigation, according to the evidence gathered by OTA (OTA, 1978a). New or developing preventive and screening technologies and new procedures are studied relatively infrequently, as are existing technologies of all types.

Earlier in the chapter, we pointed out that efficacy and effectiveness are two different concepts. These concepts are not clearly differentiated in the medical literature. In our conceptual model, all medical technologies would be evaluated for efficacy (using one or more of the techniques described above) before they come into widespread use. This would involve their being tested under the most optimal conditions possible. For example, the most skillful surgeons should be involved in a test of a surgical technique. The model does not tell us what to do to assure effectiveness. Once a technology has come into widespread use, questions are seldom raised about how it is being used. Yet use of technologies does vary substantially, and technologies are sometimes modified through use so that, in effect, they become different technologies. Coronary bypass surgery illustrates several of these problems. After its initial development, it diffused fairly rapidly. It was developed as a treatment for severe coronary disease of a life-threatening nature but, once developed, it was applied to more and more patients. Patients with angina pectoris are now commonly treated with such surgery. In addition, many surgeons whose skills are unknown are now doing the surgery. The medical literature contains virtually no analyses of the effectiveness of medical technology—that is, research on how beneficial a technology is when applied by an average practitioner in an average setting. Yet in some ways, this is the more important and interesting question. We predict that in the future this problem will be of great concern, and that the number of studies of effectiveness, now few in number, will increase.

Synthesis

Synthesis involves a critical analysis of the results of testing (available data from preclinical to clinical experience, epidemiological studies, and controlled trials) and all other available and relevant information. It often takes the form of judgments or recommendations regarding the appropriate indications for use of technology. Consensus development sometimes can be considered a synthesis activity. Syntheses are commonly found as review articles in the literature (Abrams and McNeil, 1978). However, this literature if often of poor quality (Feinstein, 1974; Fletcher and Fletcher, 1979; Gore et al., 1977; Schor and Karten, 1966) and is usually not directed toward the needs of practitioners (Williamson, 1977; Young, 1980).

Federal Government synthesis activities are expanding. The consensus development activities of NIH are too new for evaluation of their effects. The hypertension synthesis may have had positive impact. Many of the consensus exercises, however, appear to be modifications of standard seminars and conferences. How well these activities fulfill the synthesis function remains to be seen, but there is a great potential. The process by which the National Center for Health Care Technology recommends coverage decisions to Medicare may represent another synthesis activity. However, all synthesis activities are hampered by the lack of well-validated information on efficacy and safety.

Dissemination

Many of the comments relating to synthesis also apply here. The success of dissemination activities does not depend only on the distribution or publication of information, no matter how relevant or important that data may be. More critical is *effective distribution*—actually making contact with the intended audience and convincing that audience of the importance and validity of the information. Dissemination should be designed to influence behavior or at least to increase the opportunity for informed behavior change by physicians or other target populations. It is frustrating to note that little satisfactory research has been conducted on methodologies for engaging in effective dissemination or for evaluating the success of dissemination activities. Much of the research that does exist is inconclusive, and the research that is well regarded is not applied to any major degree (Health Technology Management, 1977). The quality and success of dissemination, then, are the important variables here, and the simple level of activity is merely an unsatisfactory surrogate for them.

Federal agencies have not assigned a high priority to disseminating information. FDA sometimes sends letters to all physicians as one mechanism for distributing important information. The National Center for Health Services Research (NCHSR) frequently disseminates information to a wide audience by issuing Research Reports that describe the results of projects funded or conducted by the agency. Also, NIH has provided information, primarily to the professional community, through its demonstration and control projects, through the National Library of Medicine, and through other activities, including a regular feature in the *Journal of the American Medical Association*. One of NCHCT's mandates is to coordinate and expand dissemination of relevant information. The private sector also has multiple channels that encourage the flow of information, and professional societies have been expanding their activities in this area.

Status of Efficacy and Safety Information

Based on the above evidence, we believe that there are shortcomings in the current ways in which efficacy and safety information is developed and disseminated. The data inadequacies—that are at least in part the result of the shortcomings—and the resulting inappropriate diffusion and use of technologies need examination.

Many technologies have come into widespread use before their lack of efficacy or safety was discovered. A psychosurgical procedure called leucotomy, or lobotomy, for example, was widely adopted in the early 1950s and was subsequently abandoned when its efficacy and safety were seriously challenged. The Wasserman test for diagnosing syphilis was used for more than 40 years until it was discovered that only half of the patients with positive test results actually had the disease (McDermott, 1977). More recent examples include internal mammary artery ligation (Barsamian, 1977), colectomy (surgical removal of the large intestine) for epilepsy (Hiatt, 1975), lumbodorsal sympathectomy and gastric freezing (Fineberg, 1979; Hiatt, 1975), and hyperbaric oxygen treatment for cognitive defects in the elderly (OTA, 1978a, pp. 55f.).

Questions of efficacy have been raised recently regarding a number of medical technologies currently in use (Cochrane, 1972; Frazier and Hiatt, 1978; Hiatt, 1975; Bunker et al., 1977; McDermott, 1977; OTA, 1978a, b; Fineberg and Hiatt, 1979). As mentioned earlier, only 10 to 20 percent of all procedures used in medical practice have been shown by controlled clinical trials to be of benefit (White, 1968); many of the other procedures may not be efficacious. Questions have been raised about such technological applications as oral drug treatment for diabetes (Maugh, 1975; Chalmers, 1975), respiratory therapy (Barach and Segal, 1975), oral decongestants (Lampert et al., 1975), thermography for diagnosing breast cancer (Moskowitz et al., 1976), ergotamine for migraine headache (Waters, 1970), immune serum globulin for preventing hepatitis (Seeff et al., 1977), intensive care for pulmonary edema (Griner, 1972), coronary care units (Mather et al., 1971), and radical mastectomy (McPherson and Fox, 1977).

Such widely used technologies as tonsillectomy, appendectomy, and the Pap smear have not been completely assessed for efficacy (OTA, 1978a). Others, such as electronic fetal monitoring (Banta and Thacker, 1979a) and coronary bypass surgery (Braunwald, 1977; Preston, 1977), have been diffused rapidly without careful evaluation. Concern about risks has led to questions regarding the use of mammography (Bailar, 1977) and skull x-ray.

The above are only examples. Others could be listed. Although perfect information on efficacy and safety can never be attained, shortcomings in assessment systems may be impeding a closer approximation of that goal. The status of efficacy and safety information cannot be exactly determined, but the combination of long lists of examples of technologies inadequately assessed and shortcomings in assessment processes indicates that improvement is possible.

7
Costs and Their Evaluation

> All progress is based upon a universal innate desire on the part of every organism to live beyond its income.
>
> Samuel Butler

During the 1970s much of health policy focused on rising medical costs. For 1978 national health expenditures totaled $192 billion, a sum that represented 9.1 percent of the U.S. Gross National Product (GNP) and an increase of more than 3 percentage points in GNP share since the first full year of Medicare and Medicaid in 1966 (National Center for Health Statistics, 1980, p. 244; Gibson and Fisher, 1978). Health expenditures have been rising throughout the century, but since the inception of Medicare and Medicaid there has been a decided increase in the rate of growth. Neither population growth nor the aging of the population adequately explains this increase—real, age-adjusted per capita expenditures rose 55 percent from 1965 to 1975 (Enthoven and Noll, 1979).

From one perspective, the alarm about rising medical care expenditures appears misplaced. Medicare and Medicaid have improved access to services and have increased their use by the aged and the poor. The expansion of the medical care sector, especially hospitals, has provided employment for those groups with the highest unemployment rates, namely women, blacks, and low income wage-earners (Fein and Bishop, 1976). In addition, the purpose of medical technologies is to improve patients' health. It appears inconsistent to begrudge spending for medical technologies while extolling the expansion of other sectors.

The rejoinder to this argument points out that spending for financing services (such as Medicare and Medicaid) has crowded out other health programs in the competition for limited resources. Nor has the problem of limited resources been restricted to competition among health programs.

> One researcher estimates that we are now putting tens of thousands of people in the hospital each year at a cost of $43 million to save each additional life.

The issue is not necessarily whether each life is worth $43 million, but whether many more lives could be saved for the same $43 million used more wisely. Since we as a Nation do not appear committed to meeting all of our social needs (millions are ill-fed, ill-housed, and ill-clothed), we cannot afford to ill-use our financial resources [Cooper and Gaus, 1979].

This overall social issue has many dimensions, and no apparent consensus or resolution currently exists. However, parts of the issue can be addressed. This chapter first discusses the contribution of technology to total medical expenditures and then the costs of specific technologies.

The basic question is not the absolute amount of expenditures on each technology, but whether or not the benefits of a medical technology outweigh its costs relative to alternative ways of managing a medical problem and to alternative uses of these funds. Expenditures in this chapter are considered in a descriptive sense, as the product of price charged times quantity used. Behavioral and systems explanations for the spending observed were discussed in Chapter 5.

The Role of Technology in Total Medical Expenditures

For most sectors of the economy, new technologies that are adopted and used are assumed to improve the efficiency or the quality of production. In medical care, however, the market is not necessarily a good test for the desirability of a technology. As described in Chapters 4 and 5 of this book, the medical care system may retain and encourage technologies that are neither efficacious, efficient, nor socially desirable. This fact heightens the importance of critically evaluating the effects of medical technologies.

The number of medical technologies available has mushroomed in recent years, and these new medical technologies have been cited as a major cause of rising expenditures (Gaus, 1975). Halfway technologies, which alleviate the effects of, but do not prevent or cure, disease, are usually expensive (Thomas, 1974, p. 31). The intensity of services, that is, the number of diagnostic tests and therapies provided to a patient, has also increased substantially.

Although the role of medical technology in rising expenditures has been subjected to a substantial amount of research, the results have not been definitive. Either explicitly or implicitly, most of these empirical studies have defined technology as a residual—that is, as the effect that remains after accounting for other more easily defined and measured influences, such as increases in the general price level.

Ideally, the direct and indirect effects of medical technology throughout the medical care sector would be measured. A new piece of equipment, for example, has direct expenses of operation, supplies, wages, and interest. Indirectly, a new technology may require new skills for health professionals and make old skills obsolete. It also may lead to the addition of other services, such as testing or hospitalization, and replace certain existing services. Further, it may reduce or increase the overall use of hospital and ambulatory care. Data to estimate the full effects of technology are rarely complete for a specific technology and certainly imperfect for technology overall. Resorting to the residual approach has often been viewed as the most practical expedient.

Because of data limitations, most studies of technology's effect on expenditures limit the analysis to hospitals. The possibility of detecting system-wide effects is thereby eliminated. If technology reduced the need for hospitalization, that effect would be missed in a study limited to hospitals. Such a study might even show that lengths of stay or expenditures per patient had risen if the remaining cases were more serious or more costly.

Estimates of the effect of technology on per diem hospital cost increases range from about 33 to 75 percent, depending on the definition of technology, the period of time, and method of calculation (Waldman, 1972; Feldstein and Taylor, 1977; Klarman, 1979). Dividing cost increases into price and nonprice effects, these analyses used, as a proxy for the effect of technology, the increase in costs resulting from greater use of labor and nonlabor inputs. The highest figure of 75 percent pertained to the period from 1955 to 1975, and the lower figure of 33 to 43 percent pertained to the period from 1966 to 1976.[1]

Another study identified the effect of technology as the remaining unexplained increase in hospital expenses per admission after accounting for changes in demand, case mix, and wage rates (Davis, 1974). The 38 percent attributed to technology included other undefined changes that occurred during the period under study, from 1962 to 1968.

Two studies of total health care expenditures attributed a less important role to technology. If technology reduced the amount of hospitalization, one would expect an analysis of total medical expenditures to show technology as less cost-generating (Altman and Wallack, 1979). Both Fuchs and Mushkin et al. measured technology's effect as the unexplained residual after taking account of such variables as population growth, price rises, and real income growth (Fuchs and Kramer, 1972; Mushkin et al., 1976).

---

[1] Cromwell et al. (1975) estimated the effect of one type of technology, major movable equipment, on hospital per diem costs at about 9 percent per year. This estimate pertained only to direct expendintures on equipment; the complementary inputs, such as personnel needed to operate the equipment, would add more to costs (p. 228).

For the period 1947 to 1967, Fuchs reported that technology added 0.6 percentage points to the 8.0 percent annual increase in total health care expenditures. Mushkin and associates concluded that technology reduced by 0.5 percent the 7.7 percent annual increase from 1930 to 1975. Unlike Fuchs, Mushkin et al. included a variable for the growth in third-party payments. Also important to the different results was the inclusion of the pre-war period, which captured the effect of advances such as antibiotics on the treatment of infectious diseases.

Many of the above studies of hospital and total expenditures stressed the changing nature and quantity of services provided to patients. Clearly, price and input increases were symptomatic of a changing product over the years. In fact, another approach to identifying the role of technology in rising expenditures has been to analyze the changing use of particular services or the changing pattern of testing for certain medical conditions.

Redisch (1974) found that the use of seven hospital ancillary services was responsible for about 40 percent of the increase in operating cost per patient day adjusted and in operating cost per admissions adjusted, from 1968 to 1971. The seven services were pathology tests, nuclear medicine procedures, pharmacy items, laboratory tests, diagnostic radiology procedures, therapeutic radiology procedures, and blood bank units.

Scitovsky and McCall (1976) traced the change in costs of treating 11 conditions at the Palo Alto Medical Clinic, a multispecialty, largely fee-for-service group practice. Between 1951 and 1964 the real costs of treating only two of the nine conditions studied fell: otitis media and pregnancy/delivery. From 1964 to 1971 the real cost of treating 5 of 11 conditions fell: pregnancy/delivery, breast cancer, closed reduction of children's forearm fractures with anesthetic, nonhospitalized pneumonia, and nonhospitalized duodenal ulcer. Scitovsky and McCall speculated that in numbers of cases and costs, the six conditions whose real costs rose outweighed those that were cost-saving. Those whose costs rose from 1964 to 1971 were otitis media, simple and perforated appendicitis, children's forearm fractures with cast only and with closed reduction but no anesthetic, and myocardial infarction.

The general increases in diagnostic tests and therapeutic procedures per diagnosis were especially striking. Laboratory tests per case of perforated appendicitis rose from 5.3 in 1951, to 14.5 in 1964, to 31.0 in 1971. Inhalation therapy procedures per myocardial infarction rose from 12.8 in 1964 to 37.5 in 1971.

Despite the different proxies for technology and the different approaches to measuring its effect on expenditures, certain common themes emerge from these studies. The use of technology clearly has been rising during the past two decades, and greater service intensity has contributed to rising medical expenditures. Only Mushkin and associates' study found that technology, on balance, saved costs, and their work spanned a much longer time period. Even the lowest estimates attribute one-third of the rise in *hospital* costs to technology, and the highest estimates reached as much as three-fourths of the total.

The extent of the *systemwide* effect, however, is not so clear. The two nonhospitalized conditions studied by Scitovsky and McCall (pneumonia and duodenal ulcer) experienced real cost reductions from 1964 to 1971. Unlike tests for the hospitalized conditions, diagnostic tests for these two conditions stayed constant or declined slightly. Scitovsky estimated ambulatory tests and x-rays at about $5 billion, or about 5 percent of total personal health care expenditures in 1975 (Scitovsky, 1979). To some extent, these tests may have been substituted for physician services (Scitovsky, 1979). Or, technologies may have reduced hospitalization, reduced ambulatory costs, or prevented illness (Altman and Wallack, 1979). Scitovsky as well as Altman and Wallack have called for cost studies of the most prevalent medical conditions to determine whether a few are responsible for rising expenditures or whether the effect is widespread.

The changing nature of medical care, a common theme of these studies, is both an explanation and a criticism of technology's role in rising expenditures. Early studies assumed more services were synonymous with better quality care (Scitovsky, 1967). But, as described in Chapter 6, recognition has grown that many technologies are being used extensively in situations where they may be inappropriate (OTA, 1978a). The focus, then, has shifted away from analysis of technology and medical expenditures as overall categories, to the benefits and costs of specific technologies applied in particular circumstances.

Evaluating Specific Technologies

The formal techniques of comparing costs and benefits have been applied to health programs only since the late 1950s (Fein, 1958; Klarman, 1974; Weisbrod, 1961). Benefit-cost analysis and a variant, cost-effectiveness analysis, are designed for programs that receive an insufficient evaluation in the marketplace. These complex analyses may be indicated when programs have important effects that are not reflected in market prices. Otherwise, a simple comparison of per unit costs would be a sufficient basis for decisions.

The market price may fail to reflect the full effects of using a medical technology. Unintended side effects may occur. Immunization, for example, may confer protection to the unvaccinated (herd immunity) or may cause adverse side effects in some people vaccinated. Health programs such as malaria eradication may be considered a public good, whose use and benefit for one person does not lessen its availability for others. Furthermore, social and individual valuations may differ because individuals are usually more concerned with immediate effects, while the social perspective could extend across generations.

Methodology of Benefit-Cost and Cost-Effectiveness Analyses

Both benefit-cost and cost-effectiveness analyses enumerate the implications of different programs, usually from a societal perspective. Cost-effectiveness analysis compares the use of alternative technologies to attain a common goal, such as accurate diagnosis or improvement in patient health. The cost-effectiveness ratio itself presents the net change in costs to the net change in effectiveness that results from using one technology rather than another. The methodology is still evolving (Weinstein, 1979). Costs, for example, may incorporate such expenses as those of any additional resources needed to use one technology instead of another, treatment of any side effects, savings in treating the disease, and medical services needed during any extended years of life (Weinstein and Stason, 1977; Willems et al., 1980). The goal or effect may range from greater diagnostic accuracy to improved health. The costs and effects are usually restricted to the medical care sector. On efficiency grounds, the alternative with the lowest cost-effectiveness ratio is preferable, because it could achieve a given effect at least cost. An actual decision about use, however, would incorporate other social effects, such as equity.

Benefit-cost analysis is broader in scope. Unlike cost-effectiveness analysis, the benefit-cost framework theoretically enumerates all the implications of different programs and is not limited to the medical care sector. In fact, the programs compared usually have many different effects, such as changes in mortality, disability, and working time. The common unit of measurement invariably chosen to express these different effects is dollars. Benefits are savings in the use of resources, such as costs avoided, years of life saved, and suffering avoided. Costs measure the use of resources from carrying out a program, such as treatment of side effects, use of medical personnel and supplies, and, perhaps, services needed during added years of life (Klarman, 1974). Theoretically, the alternative with the greatest net of benefits minus costs is preferred.

Some of these variables, such as treatment costs, already have dollar values. But others, notably years of life and quality of life, must have a monetary value imputed for benefit-cost analysis. Analysts often use average annual income earned, but that proxy is fraught with conceptual problems. The lives of women, blacks, retired workers, and the poor are thereby valued below those of males, whites, the employed, and the affluent. Although such weighting may reflect the realities of labor markets, it does not necessarily provide an accurate reflection of social values or an appropriate basis for public decisions. In addition, the very procedure of using income or livelihood to value lives is controversial. The value of life to an individual and to society extends beyond earning power to include subjective factors associated with the quality and meaning of life (Schelling, 1968; Acton, 1978).

To the extent that alternative medical technologies have a common outcome, cost-effectiveness analysis can be used and the problems of valuing life can largely be avoided. The common goal of health programs is to improve health status, and, in theory, a composite health status index could serve as the single goal. "Quality-adjusted life years" is such an index, wherein additional years of life are weighted according to levels of health to derive years of healthy life (OTA, 1979c; Weinstein and Stason, 1976).

In both benefit-cost and cost-effectiveness analyses, values should be discounted to give the present value of the future stream of benefits and costs. The advisability of discounting has two bases: people prefer to consume now rather than later (positive time preference) and want a reward for waiting; and funds could be invested in other projects and interest received (opportunity cost). Although they are not expressed in monetary terms, the effects in the denominator of the cost-effectiveness ratio have also been subjected to discounting (OTA, 1979c; Weinstein and Stason, 1976).

The fact that resources are limited and choices must be made among alternative and competing uses is implicit in benefit-cost and cost-effectiveness analyses. The decision rules of selecting the alternative with the highest net benefit or the lowest cost-effectiveness ratio entails the assumption that resource allocation should be based on maximizing benefits per dollar spent or on minimizing the cost of a desired outcome. In fact, choosing among alternative technologies that each have some marginal value is a growing issue in health care and health policy.

Limitations of Benefit-Cost and Cost-Effectiveness Analyses

These techniques have definite limitations. Benefit-cost and cost-effectiveness analyses do not provide the final word as to which alternative to choose. The theoretical models are inherently incomplete and the results need to be supplemented with other information for decisionmaking. Like economics itself, these techniques stress efficiency considerations. Distribution effects and equity considerations have not been well incorporated into the technique (Klarman, 1979). Fein (1977) has stressed the importance of this shortcoming:

> Yet much of society's agenda deals with equity and distribution. . . . It may be, for example, that screening is justified even if it yields a low rate of return because it reaches persons whom the private sector would otherwise neglect.

Social values, ethical considerations, and political realities may well take precedence over analytical results. Since the swine flu program in 1976, debate about a public influenza program has hinged on liability for vaccine side effects with little mention of cost effectiveness. Or, if behavioral factors, such as expected vaccination rates, are not predicted accurately, the benefit-cost or cost-effectiveness results may become invalid.

The analytical results are also biased toward factors that can be quantified (Klarman, 1974). Pain and suffering, quality of life, and equity can be noted but, if not quantified, will not appear in the numerical results. Verbal qualifications can stress the unquantifiable aspects and exclusions, but readers usually pay more attention to the statistics (Fein, 1977).

Another limitation is the need for information about the efficacy of a technology (Klarman, 1974). Lack of information about efficacy may plague analyses of technologies in use for some time. Also common is diminishing efficacy as the use of a technology, such as the stool guaiac test, is expanded by repetition on the same patients or by extension to medical conditions where its use is less appropriate (Neuhauser and Lewicki, 1976).

Accurate measurement of costs poses equally severe conceptual and practical problems. Theoretically, costs should represent the value of additional resources required for one alternative compared to another, resources that are thereby withdrawn from other potential uses. Identifying appropriate incremental costs is conceptually difficult in hospitals, for example, where facilities have multiple uses (Deane et al., 1978). Aside from the appropriate allocation of costs is the difficulty of calculating the costs attributable to a given technology (Wagner, 1979). Hospital charges or physician fees are commonly used, but may bear little relationship to true incremental costs.

Another limitation stems from the lack of a standard analytical model. Most studies differ in the variables included or technique chosen, thus inhibiting comparisons of the results. Cost-effectiveness analysis especially is still evolving, and many of the different models represent attempts to deal with conceptual problems.

A major conceptual problem for benefit-cost analyses has been valuing lives saved, as discussed above. Analysts of medical technology have increasingly turned to cost-effectiveness analysis to evaluate approaches to such conditions as influenza, end-stage renal disease, and hypertension (Klarman and Guzick, 1976; Klarman et al., 1968; Weinstein and Stason, 1976). Cost-effectiveness analysis avoids the problem of expressing a life in monetary terms. However, benefit-cost analyses, which quantify all factors in common terms, have the advantage of being comparable across and within program areas.

Refining a health status index to express the many facets of health remains a challenge for cost-effectiveness analysis. Researchers at the National Center for Health Services Research and the National Center for Health Statistics in HHS are addressing this problem (Wan and Livieratos, 1978).

The applicability of the cost-effectiveness results is restricted. Cost-effectiveness ratios may not be comparable within medical care if the effects differ. How does cost per cancer diagnosis compare to cost per heart attack victim saved? Confined to the medical care sector and expressed in health effects, cost-effectiveness ratios will not theoretically be comparable to those for other subject areas. Spending for health could not then be compared to spending for transportation or energy. In practice, these comparisons are difficult in any case.

Discounting raises problems for both kinds of analyses. Although the need for discounting is well accepted, disagreement surrounds the choice of a particular rate. Interest rates in financial markets often serve as proxies for discount rates to apply to costs. However, there is controversy about the appropriate rate for public projects. A different rate would be chosen depending on whether one stresses the concept of opportunity cost or social time preference, as described earlier. Another consideration is that society has a longer time horizon than individuals, who prefer more immediate results (social time preference). Some cost-effectiveness analyses have applied the same discount rate to effects as to costs (Weinstein and Stason, 1976; Willems et al., 1980), but neither an appropriate rate nor a reasonable proxy is clear. At present, any analysis should indicate the sensitivity of the results to alternative discount rates.

Another conceptual problem occurs in evaluating a technology with multiple uses and effects. Because pneumococcal vaccine could provide immunity against several of the pneumococcal diseases besides pneumococcal pneumonia, an analysis of pneumonia alone overestimates the cost-effectiveness ratio of the vaccine (OTA, 1979c). If pneumococcal meningitis were included, for example, vaccination costs would remain unchanged, but costs of treating pneumococcal diseases would fall, mortality would fall, and costs and morbidity from other disease would change only slightly.

Diagnostic technologies prove particularly difficult in their multiple effects. Should diagnostic accuracy be the effect evaluated or should it hinge on altered therapy or improved health? In any case the cost effectiveness of a technology must be evaluated as compared to an alternative for a particular medical problem. The cost effectiveness of a technology amenable to different uses, such as a CT scanner, will depend on the mix of conditions for which it is used (Wagner, 1979). Overall evaluations may require assuming some representative distribution of medical problems.

Data insufficiencies hamper the conduct of economic analyses. Data on the prices of specific services and expenditures for certain diseases are not readily available. Medicare carriers and intermediaries and private third-party payers individually collect such information, but do not routinely compile it or make national estimates. National surveys of medical expenditures and physicians' charges now underway could help provide these data. An interagency task force of the Department of Health and Human Services is also attempting to develop a standard methodology for estimating expenditures for certain illnesses. Such standardization would facilitate comparisons among studies. Furthermore, the magnitude of expenditures by disease could provide a basis for targeting funds to develop new technologies or to further the use of existing ones.

These estimates lack not only price data but also epidemiological data on the incidence and prevalence of a disease and its effects on mortality and morbidity. Even for pneumonia, the fifth leading cause of death, such data are incomplete (OTA, 1979c). Without such data, the effect of an interventionist technology is unclear. Methodology is also being developed at the National Center for Health Statistics and academic centers to incorporate the interactive effects of multiple causes of death into mortality data. Patients with certain chronic conditions may have a higher probability of dying from an acute illness, but current disease-specific life tables do not incorporate these relationships.

Benefit-cost and cost-effectiveness analyses necessitate predicting or simulating future events. Predictions may assume that the present situation will continue or that specified changes will occur with or without the technology under study. Rarely have these simulations been subsequently reevaluated, even though that might suggest refinements in methodology or changes in behavioral assumptions. For example, rubella vaccination was found most cost effective for 12-year-old females (Schoenbaum et al., 1976a). But recent data from Britain (Nitzkin, 1976), which adopted this policy, indicate such low vaccination rates at that age that an acceptable level of herd immunity was not achieved; thus, previous cost-effectiveness results have been called into question. It has become accepted practice for a formal analysis to include a sensitivity analysis, which varies uncertain or unknown factors over reasonable ranges to determine the effects on the results.

Analyses for Policy Purposes

Although the first analyses in the health area were connected with policymaking, widespread policy interest in these techniques is fairly recent and appears to be derived from concerns about rising medical expenditures.

Some studies, such as Fein's study on mental illness, were performed under the auspices of a task force on a particular medical problem (Fein, 1958). Several studies have illustrated public policy considerations. A benefit-cost analysis of swine flu vaccination was concluded quickly enough to demonstrate that this technique could provide timely information for decisionmaking (Schoenbaum et al., 1976b). That study also defined the parameters on which a decision should be based. In the context of national health insurance proposals, a study of repetition of stool guaiacs illustrated the diminishing return from repeated use of a medical technology (Neuhauser and Lewiski, 1976). The OTA analysis of vaccination against pneumococcal pneumonia suggested the cost effectiveness, even for the elderly, of preventive technologies usually excluded from third-party coverage (OTA, 1979c).

The cost-effectiveness analysis of end-stage renal disease therapies conducted for the Gottschalk Committee was unusual in being connected with a user (Klarman et al., 1968). The Veterans Administration's interest in renal dialysis led to the formulation of the Committee by the Bureau of the Budget. The analysis found home dialysis more cost effective than hospital dialysis, and the VA subsequently encouraged home dialysis.

The results of HHS cost-effectiveness analyses undertaken in the 1960s were at least partly implemented. The 1967 Social Security Amendments, for example, provided for the early detection and treatment of children with handicaps (Grosse, 1972).

Centers for Disease Control have shown interest in the costs and benefits of public health programs, but do not conduct complete, formal analyses (Sencer and Axnick, 1975). The Bureau of Radiological Health in the Food and Drug Administration weighs the risk of radiation exposure and the costs of altering the technical specifications of equipment to reduce those risks. However, the Bureau does not consider the use of technology beyond technical specifications. The National Center for Health Services Research has funded economic analyses of medical technologies (Schweitzer and Luce, 1978), but has done this neither systematically nor routinely.

The National Center for Health Care Technology has been given the responsibility for setting criteria and for conducting or funding cost-effectiveness analyses and technology assessments. As described in Chapter 6, the Center has coordinated with the National Institutes of Health to perform economic analyses for technologies that are the topics of Consensus Development Conferences. These current and any future activities relating to medical technologies should be a part of a coordinated system of evaluation. Chapter 6 described a process for developing and disseminating information on efficacy and safety. The same logic applies to cost-effectiveness analyses—they cannot be performed on every technology (therefore a screening, or identification, component is critical), the results must be synthesized with other information about the technology, and effective dissemination of the resultant information is essential.

The Office of Technology Assessment is conducting a major study of the implications of using cost-effectiveness analysis to evaluate medical technologies. Using case studies to illustrate specific issues of methodology and policy, the study differs from others in providing a synthesis of the advantages and disadvantages of conducting cost-effectiveness analyses and of applying the results.

Status of Benefit-Cost and Cost-Effectiveness Information

Although many studies have examined costs and effects, few have undertaken formal cost-effectiveness or benefit-cost analyses. Preventive technologies have been subjected to the largest numbers of formal analyses. Most studies of vaccines have used benefit-cost analysis and have used livelihood measures to value the morbidity and mortality averted. Studies of influenza vaccination and swine flu vaccination have found net benefits greatest for those in high-risk groups (Kavet, 1972; Schoenbaum et al., 1976b). These results confirmed the medical profession's recommendation that high-risk groups be vaccinated and suggested that targeting the vaccine to these groups could raise net benefits (Willems et al., 1980).

In general, cost-effectiveness analysis is increasingly preferred to benefit-cost analysis (Warner et al., 1979), presumably to avoid the problems of valuing life. However, major methodological problems remain and call into question the general applicability of the techniques. The formulation of the model is continuing to evolve, and may appropriately vary depending on the policy issue under study. Lack of a standard model often prevents comparisons among technologies. Diagnostic technologies pose particular problems for analysis.

Much more attention needs to be given to the implications of having and using cost-effectiveness results before analyses are performed on a wide scale. Amassing data sets and performing analyses are expensive undertakings. Cost alone indicates the necessity for criteria and priorities for conducting evaluations. But who will use the results is unclear (Luft, 1976). And how they are used could have social and ethical effects that reach far beyond cost considerations.

8
Medical Technology and Social Values

The very success of science has ended its pleasant isolation.

Robert Sinsheimer

The social implications of medical technology are often the most challenging and difficult aspects of evaluation. There are several reasons for this: it is difficult to tell in advance which of the thousands of medical technologies will have serious social implications and for whom; such impacts are difficult to identify even as they are occurring or afterwards, and even more difficult to evaluate once identified; there is less interest in this type of evaluation; and, very important, few mechanisms exist to take action based on the results of evaluation. With growing recognition of limited resources, it is obvious that more explicit attention needs to be paid to these difficult issues.

First, some terms. A societal value or social value is a concept, relationship, or institution that a society considers to be important, as expressed through that society's written and unwritten laws of behavior and responsibility. Such values can and do vary among societies and over time. Life itself is obviously an important value in our society, as demonstrated by the many proscriptive laws dealing with the socially unapproved taking of a life. Various subgroups within a society may have diverse values. Using life again as the example, consider the divergent views on abortion or capital punishment. Other examples of commonly held social values are industriousness, honesty, belief in a supernatural being (note that social values can recede in importance for significant segments of the population over time), the family, education, justice, and health. Social values encompass the ethics and morality of a society. Ethics can be viewed as a "generally shared set of felt duties, obligations, rights, ideas of justice, and of good and evil" (Behney, 1974). The ethical system of a society is its collection of and operation on moral norms, which can be thought of as survival values. That is, "all norms are system maintenance devices, but when a society believes that certain bare minima must be maintained at all costs, these rituals may be called morals" (Turney-High, 1968, p. 223). Another term of importance is ethical implication. An ethical implication of a medical technology is an impact, deriving from the actual, proposed, or potential use of a technology, that threatens one or more of society's moral norms. Social implications include ethical implications but can also include a broad array of impacts. Any impact caused by a medical technology that affects a social value significantly, including concepts, relationships, and institutions, represents a social implication.

Another term of importance is bioethics. The developing field of bioethics is a newly emerging, interdisciplinary area of inquiry concerned with the social, ethical, theological, and legal implications of advances or developments in biomedical research or technology (Fox, 1979a).

The emergence of this field is of interest to our discussion because of the interest and concerns that lie behind it. It has been only in the past 15 years that such concerns with issues related to biomedical research and medical technology have become organized and seen as legitimate (Reich, 1978). There is good evidence that a "serious reexamination of certain basic cultural assumptions on which modern medicine is premised may be taking place" (Fox, 1979b).

Clearly, the relationship between medical technology and social values is reciprocal. Just as technologies affect values, so too do social values affect medical technologies and their development, use, and evaluation (Veatch and Branson, 1976). It is not strictly possible to say that a certain effect is the result of a social value's forcing a change in the use or development of a technology as opposed to that effect's being in fact the result of a subtle change in social or cultural attitudes occasioned by a medical advance. Nevertheless, in order to perceive some order in phenomena it is often useful and possible to act as though order existed. For the purposes of discussion, then, we will suppose that at times one end of the reciprocal relationship can be said to be primary. With this in mind, some of the ways that social values affect the development, evaluation, and use of medical technology will be illustrated.

Medical technologies and their patterns of use are in a very real sense a reflection of subtle interactions among various social values: for example, the value we as a society place on health, on innovation, on financial security, on "doing things through technology." The developed countries have thus often pursued medical technology for a variety of reasons. Fuchs (1976) asked why such countries pursue national health insurance when such a policy is, in his view, economically irrational, since it encourages overuse of medical services. He noted that the drive for insurance coverage may have little to do with health: "Externalities, egalitarianism, the decline of the family and traditional religion, the need for national symbols—these all play a part. In democratic countries with homogeneous populations, people want to take care of one another through programs such as national health insurance. . . ." Fuchs could have included "faith in medical technology" as one of those factors.

Further, the definitions of health and of illness or medical conditions that shape our conception of necessary or desirable technologies are themselves expressions of social values (Fox, 1979d). The changing views of mental illness are an example. A more general example is the rapidly gained popularity of the World Health Organization's definition of health as "a state of complete physical, mental, and social well-being" (World Health Organization, 1971). Definitions like this, and more important, the cultural attitudes and social forces behind their defining, result in a widening of the scope of health conditions considered appropriate for medicine's tools. There is even a new (or newly identified) class of patients called the "worried well."

Social Values and the Development of Medical Technologies

Social values affect not only which technologies will be developed but also how such development will proceed (Beecher, 1966; Visscher, 1975). Social values, as expressed in society's concepts of health and illness, are one factor determining the research questions to be addressed. When society began to view alcoholism more as a disease than a personal failing, the search for relevant medical technologies to deal with it accelerated. It was now a "proper" medical question. Research on and development of methods to intervene in conditions of the heart were delayed for a great many years (nearly 2000) by the Judeo-Christian concept of the heart as a mystical organ containing the soul (Swazey and Fox, 1979). Another example is the birth control pill (McConnell, 1974). Although that technology is often, and appropriately, cited as one that dramatically altered social values, the necessary research and development and subsequent widespread use of the pill was facilitated by a prior and gradual shift in society's values toward contraception.

A common and significant effect that social and moral forces can exert on medical research and development may occur during the early stages of clinical investigation. If an innovation with substantial risk is at an early stage of development, the mortality or morbidity associated with its use may be quite high. Emotional and moral factors, on the part of both researchers and the public or other concerned parties, sometimes make it difficult or impossible to continue the investigations (Fox and Swazey, 1974). This may sometimes lead to a clinical moratorium. The resolution of such a moratorium or a near-moratorium will depend on a combination of medical, cultural, ethical, and personal factors (Fox, 1979e).

A note of caution: One should not conclude from the examples above that the moral norms of society are loosening. This does not seem to be the full case; certainly it is not an absolute trend. For example, many technologies have been developed using methods that would be considered unethical today. The famous gynecological surgeon of the 1800s, Marion Sims, is well known for inventing the vaginal speculum and the surgical procedure for the repair of vesicovaginal fistula. Vesicovaginal fistula is a connection between the vagina and the bladder, usually caused by physical damage during childbirth, which causes the continual leakage of urine from the vagina. Although rare, the condition was horrible. Sufferers were ostracized, primarily because of their unmistakable smell (Barker-Benfield, 1976, pp. 94–96). Sims determined to find a surgical cure for this condition. He gathered up all the women with vesicovaginal fistulae that he could find, all of them black female slaves, and operated on them repeatedly trying to find a cure. He operated without success for four years, subjecting Anarcha, one of the slaves, to thirty procedures. He was finally successful through the use of silver sutures.

Congress, influenced by, and reflecting as well as helping to form more concerned attitudes about medical experimentation, passed the 1974 National Research Act, which created the National Commission for the Protection of Human Subjects of Biomedical and Behavioral Research. The Commission investigated such issues as fetal experimentation, informed consent, and psychosurgery. Of particular note was their funding of a "Comprehensive Study of the Ethical, Legal, and Social Implications of Advances in Biomedical and Behavioral Research and Technology" (Policy Research, Inc., 1977). That study examined not only the implications mentioned in the title but also the public's understanding of such implications. The Commission now exists, with a somewhat different mission, as the President's Commission for the Study of Ethical Problems in Medicine and Biomedical and Behavioral Research.

Social Values and the Evaluation of Medical Technology

Intuitive standards of benefit and risk historically have been the guidelines for evaluation of medical technologies. This situation was partly the result of a lack of scientific methods of evaluation, but also a reflection of at least two social values: the faith that lay people placed in physicians and the related professional autonomy of medicine, and the view that medicine was in large part a personally based art of the physician. When medicine is regarded primarily as an art, population-based statistics have little relevance to the artists and their subject. This situation began to change in the late 1800s, and the pace of change has accelerated in the past few decades. Horror stories of medical quackery and the growing knowledge of lack of benefit (the therapeutic nihilism of the turn of the century) of many medical practices assaulted society's values. The resulting fear and skepticism, combined with advances in techniques to evaluate benefits and risks, led to an increase in evaluation and attempts to assure evaluation, such as the passage of the 1938 Food and Drug Laws.

Social values also affect the process of evaluation. A prime example of such forces at work is provided by the debate over the ethics of controlled clinical trials[1] (Meier, 1975; Burkhardt and Kienle, 1978; Barber, 1976; Work Group XII, 1975).

Critics of controlled trials point out that certain groups of patients have rights that are easily violated. Questions regarding the rights of children in particular are raised (OTA, 1978a, pp. 63f.). For example, when can informed consent be given by a child? At what age? With what medical conditions or illnesses? And, who, if not the child, will guard those rights? In addition, the long-term effects of treatments or other medical technology interventions can be especially serious and very long in evidencing themselves in children. Clinical trial protocols must be established with all these and more questions in mind. Similar questions may occur regarding the rights of other groups composed of convicts, the aged, and the mentally retarded, for example.

Many scientists defend the ethics of using controlled clinical trials. Some have argued that physicians cannot do just what they "believe" best; their practice must be based upon sound scientific evidence (Byar et al., 1976; Lambert, 1978, pp. 139ff.). Similarly, an honest acceptance of the fact that the relative benefits and risks of the best current therapy are not known is the first step in recognizing the need for clinical trials. If each patient is so unique as to be ineligible for statistical randomization, how can the individual physicians use clinical judgments based on past experience as the optimal guideline for determining the treatment of the next patient?

An early advocate of controlled clinical trials, Bradford Hill, wrote that:

---

[1] Also see the discussion and references in the section of Chapter 6 concerning clinical trials.

It must be possible ethically to give every patient admitted to a trial any of the treatments involved. The doctor accepts, in other words, that he really has no knowledge at all that one treatment will be better or worse, safer or more dangerous, than another. . . . If the doctor does not believe that, if he thinks even in the absence of any evidence that for the patient's benefit he ought to give one treatment rather than another, then the patient should not be admitted to the trial. Only if, in his state of ignorance, he believes the treatment given to be a matter of indifference can he accept a random distribution of patients to the different groups. . . . By certain omissions from a trial we may limit the generality of the answer given by it, but on ethical grounds that . . . must be accepted [quoted in Burkhardt and Kienle, 1978].

There are no unequivocal answers to these concerns. Certain technical improvements in statistical methods allow faster identification of intermediate results, thereby leading to sounder decisions regarding the termination date of certain types of trials. Improved consent mechanisms are being developed and could be applied more widely. Interestingly, many articles note criticisms, such as the above, about randomization but still recommend cautious use of the technique (Tancredi, 1975; Whalan, 1975).

Questions of the ethics of clinical trials change over time. For example, in the 1950s a surgical operation called internal mammary artery ligation was widely advocated by a small number of surgeons for improving blood supply to the heart. In 1958 and 1959 two randomized, controlled clinical trials were conducted by, respectively, Cobb and Diamond (Barsamian, 1977). Patients were assigned randomly to control or operative groups, and the control group was given a sham operation in which the internal mammary artery was surgically exposed, but was not ligated. Both groups of patients reported relief from anginal pain and increased tolerance of exercise. As a result of these trials, the operation was largely abandoned. Thus, the trials were of value, yet it is extremely unlikely that such a sham operation used for evaluation purposes would be considered ethical today.

So, the amount and type of evaluation of medical technologies are determined not just by scientific rationale but also by social desires and concerns. These social values often conflict. Ethical concerns sometimes act to reduce flexibility in evaluation, while at the same time economic concerns, desires to live in a safe society, and other ethical concerns about subjecting humans to unproved medical technologies tend to encourage evaluation.

Subjects of evaluation studies, especially controlled clinical trials, are, in effect, taking risks upon themselves while the rest of society shares in any benefits the studies produce in increased knowledge. Thus, by encouraging clinical trials, society is implicitly signalling its willingness to subject small numbers of people to risks, with the expectation that a greater benefit will accrue to society. Fox points out, for example, that statements about cardiac transplantation indicate that its primary justification at this time is "the new knowledge of benefit to others in our society" (Fox, 1979b). The alternative, however, is also an assault on moral norms. By not allowing evaluation studies such as controlled trials, all members of the population on which the technology in question is used would be subjected to those same risks. Such questions become particularly acute when one group, such as the poor, bears the risks of experimentation for the entire society.

Social Values and the Use of Medical Technology

Use of a technology depends on the subtle and complicated interaction of a great many forces. Some of these are medical, such as the degree to which the disease etiology is known in a specific case. Others are financial. Still others are cultural, ethical, religious, legal, or other social forces. For instance, use of diagnostic x-rays is in part determined by the physician's personal experience with or awareness of the litigation-prone nature of our society. The fear of malpractice leads to defensive medicine, which is, therefore, a socially, as opposed to medically, derived pattern of practice. This phenomenon was described in Chapter 5. Legal definitions of death and laws on organ donation and on abortion obviously affect use of technologies.

Sometimes social pressures will act in competing ways. Economic efficiencies, in theory, would act to encourage the use of home renal dialysis. Yet other social factors (in addition to the fiscal incentives inherent in present systems of financing and delivering medical care) may exert opposite pressures. In urban ghettos, for example, indigent patients living alone, in rooms without adequate plumbing or other facilities, may not be able to realize the potential benefits of home dialysis that are available to others in more comfortable situations (Fox, 1979e).

Social desires for access or equity may conflict with the desire to provide medical care rationally. Because of concerns about technology, public programs have generally moved somewhat more aggressively to evaluate medical services than have private programs. In April 1977 the Institute of Medicine, in a study commissioned by the Blue Cross Association, recommended that CT body scans be covered. Blue Cross/Blue Shield carriers moved rapidly to implement the recommendation. However, it was August 1978 before CT body scanning was covered in the Medicare program. Thus, for more than a year, elderly people covered by the Federal program had less access to CT scanning services than the general population. Whether the CT scans were necessary or not is beside the point. The desire to be certain that the services were efficacious in this case delayed the coverage decision, with serious implications for equity.

This type of mixture of medical, economic, and other social forces commonly affects decisions about technologies. Another example is the administration of rubella vaccine to children in order to produce herd immunity (LoGerfo, 1979). From a strictly medical standpoint centered on the interests of the individual patient, this is difficult to justify, due to the possibility of negative side effects without an offsetting potential direct benefit. Yet there is obviously, from the perspective of society, a collective benefit, hence the common requirement that entering school children submit proof of immunization.

The above sections set out a brief, admittedly sketchy, discussion of how social values or forces affect medical technologies. The discussion did not step too far inside the enticing morass of the philosophy of medicine in society (as exemplified by the symbolism of illness and its relation to social duty, to evil, and to magic). Issues of that type, however, tie directly into the relationships suggested here and should not be discounted.

The Assessment of Social Implications of Medical Technologies

The previous section defined social implications and discussed some of the ways the social values exert pressures on medical technologies. This and the following sections examine the reverse phenomenon. It should be kept in mind, though, that the process of assessing the impacts of medical technologies on social values and systems can also be used to examine the effects of those social values on technologies.

Nearly every technology will have some medical effect: positive, negative, or some combination of both. It is not true, however, that most medical technologies will have social implications, with the common exception of economic impacts. Nevertheless, many will have some degree of social system or value impact. A few will have substantial implications; and a still smaller number will have the potential for profoundly affecting social thought and values. Genetic manipulation,[2] the artificial heart (National Heart and Lung Institute, 1973), and technologies for behavior control (Committee on the Life Sciences and Social Policy, 1975, pp. 79–110) are examples of this last category.

[2] The Office of Technology Assessment is currently studying the implications of present and future genetics technologies.

The necessary first step in creating an effective concern for these effects and developing methods for societal response has not yet been adequately fulfilled. That is the classification and description of types of social effects. Some attempts have been made (e.g., OTA, 1976; Behney, 1976; National Heart and Lung Institute, 1973; Committee on the Life Sciences and Social Policy, 1975), but these efforts usually have been untested, undebated listings of effects or the affected parties. The medical, social science, and bioethical communities have paid little attention to this task. The scheme presented below, therefore, is based on the individual efforts mentioned above and should only be regarded as a starting point for further work.

Classes of Social Implications

Figure 8-1 illustrates a partial array of the types of social implications that may occur. It combines this listing with some of the parties that may be affected. The cells of the resulting matrix are blank, as the specific information will depend on the technology being evaluated. If, for example, a successful artificial heart were developed, a great many of the cells would indicate implications. The cell at the intersection of "legal effects" and "society in general" might show that society would be faced with potentially serious and difficult questions surrounding the definition of life.

In order to illustrate the type of information that such a matrix would contain, we have used the example of the CT scanner in Figure 8-2 (Stocking, 1978). This figure shows five sample cells of the matrix with a possible implication indicated for each. For example, one may ask if the technology has an economic effect on individuals. The CT scanner has little direct effect because of the extent of health insurance. Likewise, one may ask if the CT scanner has ethical or moral implications for particular ethnic or racial groups. In the United States, poor people will not have equitable access. The example is designed to be illustrative, not exhaustive. Depending on which technology is under study, most of the cells might contain information, and each cell might contain numerous implications.

Nature of Social Implications

The general definition of a social impact or social implication was given at the beginning of this chapter. These effects can take place when a new technology is introduced, when a technology in general use is applied to a

Figure 8-1.
A Scheme for Classifying the Effects on Society from Use of a Medical Technology.

Type of effect \ Affected parties	Individuals; patients	Family, friends	Society in general	Subgroups of society — Occupations/ industries	Ethnic, racial, or sex	Religious affiliation or beliefs	Socioeconomic status	Age groups	Ideological beliefs	Other subgroups	• • •
Economic..............	A		B	C							
Legal.................											
Political..............											
Public administrative..											
Cultural..............											
Ethical, moral.........					D		E				
Religious.............											
Health care system....											
Related tech. systems..											
Education............											
Physical environment..											
Housing, energy, etc...											
• • •											

(The letters A-E in the cells of the matrix refer to illustrative implications of the CT scanner, which are presented in figure 8-2.)

SOURCE: Office of Technology Assessment.

Figure 8-2.
Examples of Social Implications, Based on the Impact of the CT Scanner.

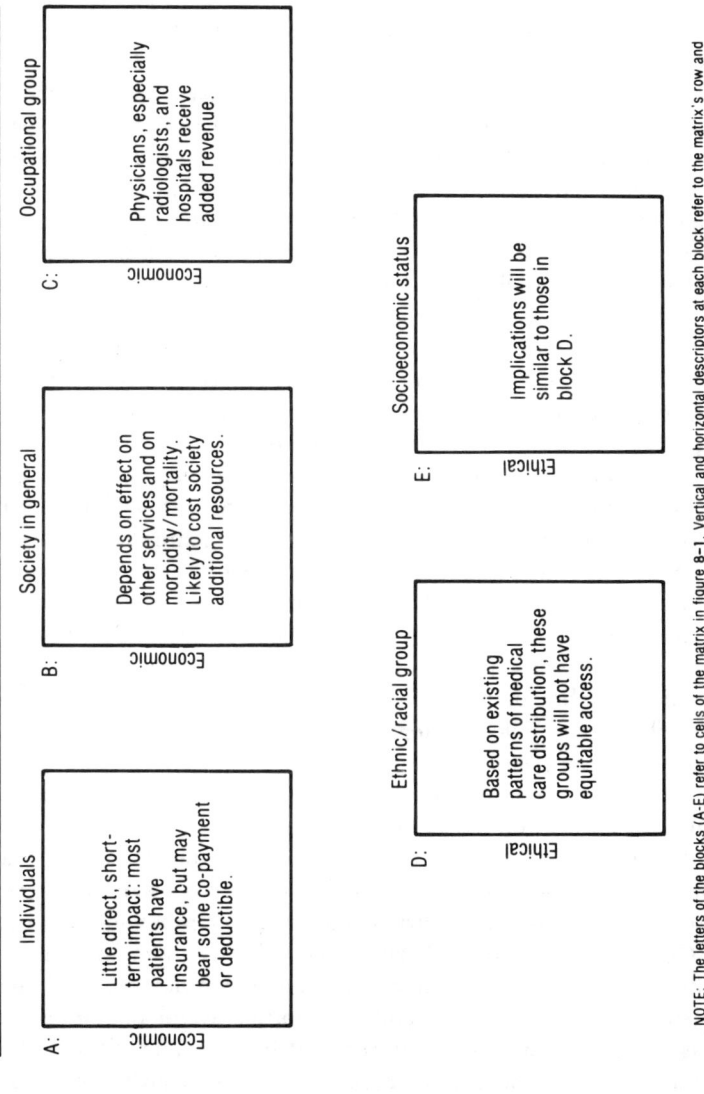

NOTE: The letters of the blocks (A-E) refer to cells of the matrix in figure 8-1. Vertical and horizontal descriptors at each block refer to the matrix's row and column headings. The possible social implications given are meant to be merely illustrative—not exhaustive—and are not the result of a full assessment.

SOURCE: Office of Technology Assessment.

different purpose, or when a technology's use even for the same purpose is significantly increased. It is possible for a technology to have social effects in advance of its introduction: witness the reexamination of scientific research and community control of research within its borders that took place before, but in anticipation of, certain high-risk recombinant DNA experiments.

Just as with efficacy and safety, a social impact can be characterized best by specifying certain aspects of the effect. The most obvious of course is *the nature of the effect itself*. For example, a change in societal sex ratios, an increased amount of adolescent sexual activity, and an unresolved legal and moral confusion over the definition of life or death are examples of effects that might be due to the widespread or emerging use of certain medical technologies. Beyond the effect itself, however, are other issues. What individuals or groups are affected? Which beneficially? Which negatively? (For these may often be different groups.) In other words, how are the social impacts distributed across society? Another issue to be addressed if social implications are to be adequately characterized is that of the conditions giving rise to the effect. These conditions are of at least two general types: technological and societal. The identified effects will depend on the way in which the technology is used. Thus, without describing the patient population, the type of delivery system, the exact nature of the technology, the extent of use, and so on, it is difficult to feel that one has described an effect understandably. Similarly, the conditions of the society that led to or were necessary for the occurrence of the specific effect should be specified. As a corollary to these specifications, it would be valuable to specify these aspects of the technology or society that, if manipulated, could heighten its positive effects or ameliorate negative consequences.

An interesting and often confounding aspect of social implications is that they may be direct or indirect effects, may occur in the short or the long run, may be intended or unintended. So far, that is similar to most types of effects—e.g., efficacy, safety, and economic. However, one difficult characteristic of social effects is that they may occur as the result of other social effects, which in turn are the result of other social effects, and so on. Obviously these are indirect effects. They are sometimes referred to as higher order effects. For instance, one first order effect of the birth control pill was contraceptive ability. Another would be serious medical complications. A second order effect might be loosening of the tie between women and the child-bearing function. A still higher order effect might be increased participation of women in the labor market. Another, more speculative, higher order effect might be a gradual shift in the attitude (or in the ability to rationally claim the attitude) that women are poor hiring prospects because "they'll just get pregnant." And so on. As another example, higher order effects of amniocentesis might include a heightening of the abortion controversy, concerns about the duty of parents to deformed or restricted-function children, and the possibility of altering the ratio of males to females in society.

Obviously, technologies and implications do not relate in a one to one fashion, or as exclusive cause and effect. The use of a technology may contribute to an effect or may detract from it. Any ultimate effects will be the result of a number of technological and social variables.

One type of social implication should be mentioned both because of its importance and because it may serve as a useful illustration. Medical technologies and their patterns of use can have important implications for access to and distribution of medical care services. Impacts in these areas can, in turn, have substantial equity implications. The CT scanner, as mentioned above, has diffused in a rather distinct pattern. While almost 20 percent of scanners are located in physician offices, very few are in large, urban public hospitals (Banta, 1980; OTA, 1980). This creates an imbalance of distribution and inequitable access to the scanners for poor people, who often receive most of their medical care in public hospitals. To a significant extent, any technological advance is fed into a delivery system that historically discriminates (for a variety of cultural, financial, and even geographical reasons), in terms of access and distribution, against poor people, minorities, the aged, and other groups. Thus, technological advances can be in part the cause of, in part the catalyst, and in part the mechanism for continued inequities.

Techniques for Assessing Social Implications

In a 1976 report, the Office of Technology Assessment suggested a number of questions that could be asked regarding a medical technology and its effects. Before discussing the possible assessment techniques themselves, we will present some of those questions (OTA, 1976, pp. 31–41). The list is illustrative and not by any means exhaustive.

> What are the medical aims, technical characteristics, and developmental state of the technology in question?
>
> What medical problems is the new medical technology designed to solve, and how severe are these medical problems: Does it diagnose an early form of the disease? Does it make diagnosis more reliable or valid? Does it treat a life-threatening symptom or syndrome? Does it correct an incapacitating but nonlethal condition?

Is the technology a major or minor innovation? Will it radically alter medical practice or will it modify and improve established procedures?

How soon can development and adoption of the new technology be expected if there are no interventions in the normal processes of research, development, testing, marketing, diffusion, and use?

How effective is the procedure? Has its medical efficacy been assessed yet? How will medical efficacy be assessed? Are rigorously controlled clinical trials possible? Underway? If controlled trials are not possible for technical or ethical reasons, is there any other way to insure that the technology is medically effective? What are the potential or proved dangers of the technology to individuals using it?

What are the implications of the technology for the patient?

What will be the quality of life of the patient who has been treated? Normally active? Moderately restricted? Physically crippled?

What psychological effects can be anticipated? Guilt? (Because of high financial and social costs to family, etc.) Anxiety? Feelings of dehumanization? Dependency?

What are the implications for the patient's family?

What will be the costs to the family? How will the new technology affect family structure? Will there be any physical dangers to the immediate family? Will the device or procedure be psychologically acceptable to the family? Will active cooperation or assistance of family members be necessary on a continuing basis? How will the new technology affect individual or family budgets?

What are the implications for society in general?

Will the new technology change the demographic characteristics of the society? For example, can changes in sex ratios or age distribution in the population be anticipated? Will the new technology affect reproductive capability of patients and thus change the genetic pool and the prevalence of genetic disease?

Will use of the new technology by an individual create threats to the environment that are properly the concern of the entire society?

Will introduction of the new technology challenge important beliefs and values of the society about birth, gender, bodily integrity, personal identity, marriage and procreation, respect for life, right to live, right to die, responsibility for each other? Will introduction of the new technology result in changes in these values?

Will the technology alter any basic institutions of society (e.g., schools, recreational facilities, prisons)?

What are the implications for the legal and political systems?

Will problems of justice, access, or fairness arise? Will they lead to litigation?

Will the manufacturer be liable for damages resulting from failure of the technology? Will liability extend only to damage to the individual or will it cover environmental effects as well?

Will use of the new technology require changes of the definitions of death or suicide?

What are the implications for the economic system?

What is the projected or present overall monetary cost of adopting the new technology?

Will income maintenance be required for those using the technology? What are the implications for programs of disability or life insurance? Pension funds? The Social Security System?

Who will pay? Who can be expected to pay? Will government support be required for development and/or use of the new technology?

How will the technology affect the national economy? Will development and use produce jobs? How will this affect overall productivity? Will the tax structure and rates be affected?

If an analyst or policymaker was interested in only one type of impact, relatively narrow forms of evaluation such as economic impact studies, cost-effectiveness analyses, decision analyses, environmental impact analyses, or the like could be undertaken (Arnstein, 1977). Broader types of analysis could draw upon systems analysis, operations research, or an emerging field called, appropriately enough, social impact assessment. Perhaps a better approach, when the effects or even the possible types of effects are unknown or highly uncertain, is to start from the perspective of technology assessment. Technology Assessment (TA) is, at least in the medical area, now more commonly known as "comprehensive technology assessment", because of the trend toward using the former term to refer to any form of evaluation of medical technologies. For our present purposes, however, we shall use technology assessment to mean "the systematic study of the effects on society that may occur when a technology is introduced, extended, or modified, with special emphasis on the impacts that are unintended, indirect, and delayed" (Coates, 1971).

Technology Assessment

Technology assessment is, in essence, simply a broader form of policy research than is commonly conducted. The goal of technology assessment, as of all policy research, is to provide decisionmakers with information on policy alternatives, such as allocation of research and development funds, formulation of regulations, or development of new legislation (Hetman, 1973; OTA, 1976; Arnstein and Christakis, 1975). Technology assessment has several features that distinguish it from other ways of examining the societal impacts of a proposed new technology. Some of the most important features of technology assessment are:

1. Technology assessment is based on an explicit analytic framework, which is specified before the study begins. Although this framework may be modified as the study proceeds, its existence helps to ensure that the implications of introducing a new technology will be systematically identified and examined.
2. It is comprehensive in scope, examining impacts on ethical, legal, and other social systems, and it considers "higher order impacts" (that is, impacts of the impacts).
3. It is carried out by a multidisciplinary group, because it requires wider expertise than any individual or single disciplinary group could be expected to possess.
4. It explicitly identifies the groups that will be affected by the proposed technology and evaluates the impacts of the technology on each party.

A comprehensive technology assessment, which can cost hundreds of thousands of dollars and last for more than a year, cannot be performed for each developing technology. It is possible, however, to perform limited assessments, either in preparation for or in lieu of efforts on a larger scale. These are also a number of less comprehensive assessment methods that might precede, be included in, or take the place of a complete technology assessment; such analyses are sometimes called partial technology assessments.

Too few technology assessments have been completed to know how the information they elicit and the recommendations they propose will be used. Furthermore, even when more assessments are available, their uses will vary with their scope and quality as well as with a variety of other endogenous factors, including political considerations and the institutional setting of the group performing the assessment.

Two possible outcomes are frequently predicted (and sometimes feared). One is that nothing will happen. The assessment may fail to identify workable policy changes. Alternatively, the results of the assessment, however solid and well documented, may be overshadowed by political, economic, or other considerations.

The second predicted outcome is that development of the technology will be blocked. The assessment may find sufficient unintended or unanticipated consequences of the new technology to justify termination of all programs for its development.

Between these two extremes, however, are a large number of possible outcomes of technology assessment that might modify relevant policy in other ways (Banta and Sanes, 1978a). Assessment might reveal how the technology could be applied in new or expanded ways. Or the development or use of the technology might be expedited, as new, unanticipated benefits are described by the assessment. When the assessment provides information to parties at interest, including the developers, these data could be used as development and implementation proceed (such as reimbursement schemes). An assessment may reveal better ways to implement (or develop) the technology in an incremental fashion. For example, limited experimental programs for its use might profitably precede large-scale implementation in some cases. In others, ways to develop and test parts of the new technology might be devised, instead of adopting an all-or-nothing approach (e.g., a left-ventricular assist device, instead of a totally implantable artificial heart).

If potential drawbacks to the new technology are identified but cannot be adequately evaluated, the assessment could stimulate research aimed at a better understanding of such risks. If negative factors can be predicted with some confidence, an assessment could lead to programs aimed at developing alternative forms of technology that would minimize these effects and maximize the benefits. When the risks are intrinsic to the technology in question, but the benefits are sufficiently large, assessment could recommend the development of programs to counteract or correct the difficulty.

An assessment could reveal the need for new controls or regulations that would be related to the development or use of the new technology. Agencies or legislative bodies could use the results of the assessment in considering whether new regulations, taxes, prohibitions, or laws would be socially desirable. In many cases, assessment could reveal the consequences of the new technology but still not be able to evaluate their importance. Programs of continued surveillance might then be instituted to monitor the development and implementation of the technology so as to ensure that appropriate information would be available to the responsible parties in a timely fashion. And if the uncertainty about the negative consequences of a new technology were sufficiently great, or if it became difficult to balance large benefits and drawbacks, the assessment could lead to a delay in the development or use of the technology until more information was gathered or until the public's response could be measured. These moratoria, whether short or long, formal or informal, could provide an alternative to a policy of continuation that would be wasteful, costly, or politically impossible to terminate at a later stage.

Current Assessment Activities

Only two Federal agencies are charged with performing broad studies of the social implications of medical technologies. One is the Office of Technology Assessment; the other is the new National Center for Health Care Technology.

Office of Technology Assessment

The Office of Technology Assessment (OTA) is an advisory arm of the United States Congress. It was authorized in 1972, funded in late 1973, and began full operations in 1974. Its basic function is to help the legislature anticipate and plan for the consequences of technological applications, and to examine the ways, expected and unexpected, in which technology affects peoples' lives. Assessments of health-related technologies have been conducted by OTA since its inception. The Health Program has issued reports on such topics as drug bioequivalence, medical information systems, carcinogenesis testing technologies, saccharin, vaccine policies, and the CT scanner. Studies on generic issues related to social impacts, efficacy and safety, and cost-effectiveness have also been conducted. Appendix A lists and briefly describes the completed studies of the OTA Health Program. The Division of Health and Life Sciences of OTA also includes a program that assesses genetics technologies and issues relating to technologies and world population, and one dealing with food, including public health nutrition, and renewable resources.

OTA is a small agency with limited personnel and financial resources.

For that reason it has concentrated its efforts on examination of either generic technological issues (such as evaluation) or on case studies from which further research questions or generalizable lessons can be gained.

National Center for Health Care Technology

This new National Center (NCHCT) has been described in Chapter 6. As mentioned there, the agency is too young to have any characterizable methods of operating. It has, however, been given a legislative mandate to conduct and support evaluations of the ethical, social, and economic implications of medical technologies. As of this writing, the NCHCT had not completed any such evaluations. A comprehensive study was being planned on maternal serum alpha-fetoprotein screening. That assessment would include examining efficacy, safety, costs, and social impacts.

Other Activities

The National Science Foundation (NSF) has been active in the area of technology assessment and has funded several studies related to health. For example, the NSF supported a comprehensive Study of Life-Extending Technologies, which identified a wide range of social impacts that might result from such technologies (Futures Group, 1977). Other Federal agencies include the National Academy of Sciences and the National Center for Health Services Research. Also, the Health Resources Administration (of HHS), which administers the National Health Planning and Resources Development Act of 1974, has become interested in technology-assessment-related issues. That Act directs the national advisory council to address, among other things, the implications of new medical technology for the organization, delivery, and equitable distribution of health care services. The National Council for Health Planning and Development has, therefore, formed a subcommittee to examine these concerns.

The private sector has some degree of interest in assessment of broad social impacts, but, except where funded by the Federal Government, this interest has not resulted in much activity. The exceptions to the above are the concerns with the ethical and the economic implications of medical and health-related technologies. The emergence of bioethics has been mentioned above. Private sector organizations include the Hastings Institute, the Kennedy Institute of Georgetown University, and the Society for Health and Human Values in Philadelphia.

Status of Social Impact Information

There is no way to adequately characterize the status of information on social impacts. Consciousness of medical technology's potential for creating positive and negative social implications has almost certainly been heightened in the past 10 years, as is obvious from media attention to the Quinlan case (Kron, 1975; Sullivan, 1975). Yet, with the exception of the rather special case of economic implications, there is very little research-derived, organized knowledge on social impacts of medical technologies. We should not hope for the same type of knowledge, and certainly not expect the same possibilities for taking actions, with general social impacts as we do for efficacy and safety or costs. Information on actual, possible, or potential social impacts would serve to open and structure public debates. It would add another dimension to public policy, but only rarely would it, by itself, determine policy (Coates, 1972).

Social aspects of a technology's development and use have sometimes been perceived as significant and occasionally have played a role in decision-making. The passage of the end-stage renal disease program under Medicare was in part a reaction to the moral issues involved. Debates about such issues as contraceptive technologies for teenagers, genetic manipulation, and psychotherapy have included strong elements of social, especially ethical, considerations.

Thus, social impacts are not entirely new to policy formulation. Our concern, though, is that very little effort has been made to systematically identify which medical technologies might have significant social impacts, to evaluate those impacts, or to synthesize and disseminate the resultant information. In the absence of this more rigorous approach, social impacts have been taken into account in policy when they have been extremely obvious and, usually, when it is very late in the diffusion process. More subtle, but perhaps more important, effects may be missed. Or, it may be too late to avoid usage or development patterns that fostered any negative impacts or to emphasize those that could have resulted in positive ones.

There has been so little experience in the medical care area with assessing social implications that it is impossible to suggest what level of effort is needed. Other than suggesting that the extremely limited resources now being devoted to it could reasonably be expanded somewhat, we can only hope that the continuing experience of OTA, NCHCT, and other organizations will provide an indication of what policymaking benefits could potentially accrue with a larger effort.

9
Assuring the Quality of Medical Care

> But every experiment is long and difficult, and the laborers are few, and the number of facts which we require to predict, enormous.
>
> Henri Poincaré

The quality of medical care provided in the United States has become a prominent policy issue for several reasons. A number of studies have shown questionable or poor quality of medical care provided in different settings to different subsets of the population, and some have even questioned whether more care improves health. Concern also exists that appropriate use be made of the latest medical technologies. Another reason is public dissatisfaction with the quality of care, especially as indicated by a rising rate of malpractice suits. But certainly driving the issue is the concern for the rapidly rising costs and the misgivings that much of the discretionary use of technologies may add little to patients' welfare or even harm it.

In this book, we have focused on two issues: (1) factors that have led to our present situation, with its large research establishment, specialty-oriented medical care system, large industry involvement in the production of medical technology, and multiple incentives for the use and overuse of medical technologies, and (2) methods for evaluating technologies so they may be more appropriately used. This chapter discusses methods of evaluating the use of medical technologies. As the science of evaluation develops, the methods of assessing quality of care will also improve. So in a sense, this chapter brings together the two themes of the book. Without valid and reliable methods of assessing quality of care, quality assurance will not be possible.

Concern for quality is not new, and has focused mainly on what physicians do. Physicians' positions give them power over others—the power of dangerous and beneficial drugs and procedures, the power to seek intimate and sensitive information, the power to advise and prescribe. Such powers may be and have been abused, often unintentionally. The same applies, but with less force, to other health workers. As government has become more and more involved in the medical care system, the goal of *assessing* quality is not sufficient. The government endeavors to protect the public. One method of doing that is through quality *assurance* programs. The PSRO program described in this chapter is an important example.

Conceptual Approaches to Quality

The term quality implies a degree of excellence. To measure such excellence, a standard of comparison must exist and a method of measurement must be available. Principles are not hard to develop. The Committee on the Costs of Medical Care published a classic statement on the quality of care that is still pertinent today, almost 40 years later (Lee and Jones, 1933, pp 6–10). Eight articles of faith were described: scientific basis for medical practice; prevention; consumer-provider cooperation; treatment of the whole individual; close and continuing patient–physician relation; comprehensive and coordinated medical services; coordination between medical care and social services; and accessibility of care for all people. These broad goals are unarguable, but they also illustrate the difficulty of assessing or even discussing all aspects of quality. Measurement is a major problem in quality assessment. The field is still new and underdeveloped, although it is developing rapidly.

Measurements of the quality of care have been used since the beginning of medicine. The Code of Hammurabi in Babylon dictated that a physician's hands might be cut off if a patient died under his care (Sigerist, 1970, p. 308), and the Hippocratic Oath stated certain standards of quality.

Criteria for medical performance emerged as medicine developed scientifically and as data were collected. Medical guilds upgraded their requirements for membership from the eighteenth century, first to require apprenticeship and then training within formal schools. In 1858 a major step occurred when Britain established one national licensing authority and made it a legal offense for anyone to falsely assume the title of medical practitioner. Quality was thus defined in terms of education received. This type of structural assurance is still common.

Methods of Defining and Assessing the Quality of Care

The literature on quality of care is extensive, and gradually a consensus has begun to emerge about how assessment can be done. Nonetheless, a confusing array of approaches and philosophies still characterizes the field. In large measure, quality assessment entails evaluating medical care on the basis of effects described in the first half of this book, especially for efficacy, safety, and social effects.

Approaches to quality assessment may be thought of as either general or specific (Jonas, 1977). General approaches examine the ability of an individual or institution to meet certain standards. Individuals are usually measured in terms of experience, education, and knowledge. Institutions are evaluated on the basis of physical structure, administrative and staff organization, minimum services, and personnel qualifications. The general approaches used in the United States are licensing, accreditation, and certification.

Specific approaches to quality measurement and control examine specific interactions of providers and patients. The major specific approaches used in the United States are hospital medical staff review committees, research studies, Professional Standards Review Organizations (PSROs), patient satisfaction, and malpractice litigation. Patient satisfaction and malpractice will not be discussed in this chapter. Others have considered the consumer's role in some detail (Institute of Medicine, 1976).

The Castonguay Commission of the Government of Quebec (1970) recognized the difficulty of formulating an operational concept of quality:

> Thus, developing a definition which reconciles all aspects or the majority of aspects of quality is, we believe, an undertaking doomed to failure. The terms of a general definition are too vague to allow scientific evaluation. On the other hand, choosing among the possible definitions of the quality of care leads to rejecting part of reality and to reducing the meaning of quality to one or some of its dimensions.

Because of this argument, the Commission did not attempt to define quality. It described quality as viewed by producers, consumers, and society. Producers evaluate professional competence and the technical quality of services and methods used, but pay little attention to access or distribution of care. The Commission felt that consumers focus on ease of access, continuity and humanization of care, and prevention of disease. Society, it felt, evaluated care as to its effect on standards of health of the population and as to whether its efficiency conforms to society's priorities (Willems, 1976).

Donabedian (1969, pp. 2–3) provided the generally accepted classification of techniques when he used the terms structure, process, and outcome. As he points out, evaluating *structure* requires the acceptance of two assumptions: that better care is more likely to be provided when better qualified staff, better physical facilities, and so forth are employed; and that we know enough to identify what is good in terms of staff, physical structure, and organization. *Process* is the evaluation of the actual activities of providers, but requires specifying which activities are appropriate. Assessment of *outcomes* is the evaluation of end results of health care in terms of health and satisfaction.

It is worth emphasizing that a variety of outcomes is possible, and more than the avoidance of death is involved. Donabedian included recovery and restoration of function as well as survival. He considered outcomes "the ultimate validators of the effectiveness and quality of medical care" but also emphasized their limitations (1966). Outcomes depend both on available knowledge and the extent to which that knowledge has been applied. Most medical practices can only be expected to apply knowledge. Evaluation of quality by outcomes requires holding constant other factors that affect outcome. This may prove difficult in studies over long periods of time, which are often necessary to discern the effects of medical care on outcomes.

Evaluating process is easier, but it produces less definitive estimates. The basic problem is described in Chapter 6: the often indeterminate relationship between standard medical procedures and favorable outcomes on health. There are two problems in establishing the relationship. The first is knowing whether physicians follow currently accepted medical procedures in their practices. In other words, are they using technologies effectively? The second is establishing the effect on outcomes under ideal circumstances, that is, efficacy.

In all three techniques, criteria are used in the evaluation process. These criteria can be either explicit or implicit. If explicit, they are written down. If implicit, they exist only in the mind of the evaluator. Evaluators are chosen because of their qualifications and reputations. All of these approaches are hampered by lack of knowledge of the value of specific interventions or technologies. Thus structure, process, and outcome have not been correlated to indicate which aspects of each are important to evaluate.

Quality Assurance Activities and Programs

Quality assurance activities depend on information on quality. A point sometimes overlooked is that assessment largely occurs in the course of attempting to control quality. As a result, most meaningful assessment is being done in mandated assurance programs with little input from philosophers and researchers on quality of care. In a sense, that is analogous to the situation described in Chapter 6: researchers produce material on efficacy and safety, but, as described in Chapter 5, it does not seem to greatly influence provider's behavior. In another sense, of course, it is quite different. The operational quality assurance activities often involve physicians' assessing their own work, and there is an assumption that that assessment assures quality. Finally, any assurance program depends on the validity of the assessment methods and the assumptions about validity that are made.

The sections that follow will give an overview of quality assurance activities.

General Approaches to Quality of Care Assessment and Control

LICENSING. Licensing systems exist in the United States for both individuals and institutions. Approximately 25 health professions and occupations are licensed in one or more states (Pennell and Stewart, 1968) and approximately 10 types of health facilities are licensed (Hollis, 1968, p. 1). Licensed health workers include physicians, osteopathic physicians, chiropractors, dentists, nurses, optometrists, pharmacists, and psychologists. Licensed institutions include hospitals, nursing homes, homes for unwed mothers and dependent children, and psychiatric hospitals and homes for the mentally retarded.

The two types of licensure have important similarities and some important differences (Jonas, 1977). Both use structural standards for measurement and both avoid evaluating discrete services. Both involve government authority and are backed by force of law. Licensing is considered to be a "police power," and thus is reserved to the states by the Constitution. Both types of licensure involve heavy input from nongovernment practitioners and professional associations, particularly physicians. Medical licensure is generally done by boards of physicians. One important difference is that individual licensure is generally for life, while institutional licensure is usually for a set time period. Licensing may be used to restrict entry to practice, and has criminal sanctions for those who practice without a license.

Medical licensure and other types of individual licensure are usually achieved by offering an examination to individuals who meet minimum educational requirements. A recent trend has been to require relicensure as a method of assuring competence. While no states require a relicensing examination, at least 23 states now require continuing medical education for reregistration of the license to practice medicine.

Institutional licensure is done by state government departments and is not dominated to the same degree by physicians. The criteria used include such factors as the ownership and auspices, the space and physical layout, the presence or absence of certain facilities and equipment, and the composition of boards of trustees.

ACCREDITATION. Accreditation is another method of quality assurance commonly used in the United States. It is used only for institutions and programs, and is generally voluntary. Groups of like institutions and organizations get together, form an organization, establish standards, and inspect and accredit programs and institutions periodically (Jonas, 1977).

Accreditation involves primarily the use of structural criteria. The criteria are similar to those used in licensing, but since accreditation often deals with educational programs, the criteria often include attention to the details of the curriculum.

Although accreditation is theoretically voluntary, it often is equivalent to licensing. For example, the Medicare law restricts payments that may be made to unaccredited hospitals, and states generally require graduation from an accredited medical school as a prerequisite to medical licensing.

Probably the most important accrediting body is the Joint Commission on Accreditation of Hospitals (JCAH). The JCAH functions as generally described above, to do periodic accreditation of hospitals. Another important accreditation mechanism is that by which medical schools are accredited (Jonas, 1977). Questions of validity have repeatedly been raised about the structural standards used in these processes (Jonas, 1977).

CERTIFICATION. Certification is a voluntary method of assuring quality of individual health workers. Standards of training and experience are applied, followed by an examination to determine qualification. Although voluntary, there are many incentives to become certified. For example, many school districts will hire only certified speech therapists. Physician specialists are certified by specialty boards made up of the specialists themselves, based on a certifying exam. All specialty boards have established policies to provide recertification of specialists as a method of assuring continued competence.

Specific Approaches to Quality of Care Assessment and Control

HOSPITAL MEDICAL STAFF REVIEW COMMITTEES. The JCAH requires that the hospital medical staff be organized to provide for committees that review at least the following: the quality of physician care; the products of surgical operations; deaths; the utilization of hospital services; the use of medical consultation services; and the general operations of all hospital divisions (Jonas, 1977). These committees deal, where appropriate to their purpose, with discrete patient care or support services. These are so-called peer-review committees.

Utilization review was mandated in the original Medicare law in 1965 as a cost-control measure. Norms were to be established for the length of stay in the hospital for most common conditions. If the review committee decided that the length of stay was not justified in a particular case, Medicare would not pay for the extra days. How this system worked is not known in detail (Ellwood, 1973, p. 31). It did, however, form a base for the Professional Standards Review Organizations (PSROs), described next.

The PSRO Program

The EMCRO Program

During the 1960s, as the cost and quality of medical care were increasingly debated, the possibility of more involvement of practicing physicians in review procedures was discussed. Of particular interest was the possibility that if inefficient use of hospitals and unnecessary operations could be prevented, money could be saved to improve other important services, such as ambulatory care and preventive medicine. Brook and Williams (1976) summarized the questions being asked: "What if practicing physicians were given the responsibility and authority to use a peer review mechanism to control both the cost and quality of care? Would this mechanism improve the quality of care given to a defined population? Would costs be at least partially contained?"

The Experimental Medical Care Review Organization (EMCRO) program was begun in 1970 by the Department of HEW (now HHS) to test this approach. The predecessor of the EMCRO program was the Foundation for Medical Care, areawide associations of physicians. Eight original EMCRO projects were funded, including projects in New Mexico and Utah. The EMCROs used various methods to review quality and contain costs, including review of medical records; claims review; definition of disease-specific process and outcome criteria and standards; preadmission certification for admission to institutions; concurrent review; and retrospective denial of payment for services. The EMCRO program was not carefully evaluated—studies tended to be inconclusive and controversial (Brook and Williams, 1976). Nonetheless, the EMCRO program became the model for the PSRO program, and a number of the EMCROs became PSROs. The impact of the EMCRO program on those who visited and observed specific programs was direct. The staff of the Senate Finance Committee, which developed the original PSRO bill, was especially affected. It is also no accident that one of the most successful EMCROs was in Utah, the state of Senator Bennett, the bill's sponsor.

Development of the PSRO Program

The PSRO program was established in 1972 by Public Law 92-603 and is administered by the Health Care Financing Administration of the Department of HHS. The purposes of the program are to help improve the quality and control the costs of medical services reimbursed through Federal payment programs. The program operates by setting standards and criteria for the desired level and quality of medical services and by evaluating against these standards the services actually provided. This process is designed to ensure that payment will be made only when services are medically necessary.

According to the Congressional Budget Office (1979), regulation of medical practice, such as that done by PSROs, is designed to alter the array of medical services delivered to patients, that is, to affect technological change. Given a standard of desirable care, a service may be inappropriate for one or more of the following five reasons:

1. Additional services could significantly improve the patient's prognosis;
2. A different course of treatment could improve the prognosis;
3. Some services are deemed "unnecessary" because they offer little if any improvement in prognosis;
4. Some services actually risk harming the patient while offering little medical benefit; and
5. Services delivered in a lower-cost setting (such as in a nursing facility, or at home) can be as effective as in a hospital [p. 4].

Obviously, determining that a service is inappropriate requires a great deal of knowledge about the efficacy of the interventions considered.

The PSRO program is based on the concepts that medical professionals are the most appropriate people to evaluate the quality of medical services, and that effective peer review at the local level is the soundest method for ensuring the appropriate use of medical care resources and facilities (Office of Planning, Evaluation, and Legislation, 1977). It may also rest on a recognition that this is politically the only feasible approach. The PSRO program is made up of separate and independent organizations covering 203 geographic areas. Each PSRO must be substantially representative of all practicing physicians in an area. The PSRO program is not yet fully implemented. In March 1977, of the 203 PSRO areas, only 120 PSRO agencies had been funded; 100 were in "conditional" status; 20 were in "planning" status. By April 1979, the areas had been consolidated to number 195. Of these, 182 had PSROs in "conditional" status, and 13 were being planned or were inactive.

PSROs usually review only services reimbursed through Federal payment programs, Medicare and Medicaid,[1] whose coverage policies and eligibility requirements are set nationally, and PSROs must function within those limits. A service may be ruled ineligible for coverage either nationally or locally, with national decisions taking precedence. Questions about coverage can be answered locally or referred to the national level for resolution. If a PSRO disagrees with coverage policies or eligibility requirements, it may ask for reconsideration of such policy. Although no such question has yet come to the national level, this mechanism does have promise as a method of obtaining reactions to the national Medicare program from the local level and from medical practitioners.

Each state with three or more PSROs has a statewide Professional Standards Review Council. Among other duties, these Councils have the responsibility to disseminate information and data among the PSROs within the state. At the national level, a National Professional Standards Review Council is established by law. According to Public Law 92-603, this Council has several functions, including one to "provide for the development and distribution, among Statewide Professional Standards Review Councils and Professional Standards Review Organizations of information and data which will assist such review councils and organizations in carrying out their duties and functions." Such information is specified as including regional norms and standards. Local PSROs are not required to accept model standards issued by the National Council. However, the National Council has authority to disapprove local standards that deviate from model standards if the Council determines that the differences are not medically justified. The National PSRO Council has provided general guidance and sample criteria sets developed by several organizations, including the American Medical Association, under contract with the Department of HHS. The purpose of these contracts has been mainly to develop criteria on medical necessity for hospitalization for different disease categories. The Health Standards and Quality Bureau (HSQB), which administers the

---

[1] Although the law mandates review of publicly funded services only, some PSROs have begun to review privately funded services also. PSROs also have authority over other health programs authorized by the Social Security Act, including Maternal and Child Health programs. Because of the small size of such programs, they will not be referred to further.

PSRO Program, hopes that both technical assistance and norms and standards will have an important educational effect, as well as affect practice directly through reimbursement policy.

Each PSRO is initially limited to reviewing hospital inpatient services. After a PSRO has demonstrated its effectiveness, the Secretary of HHS may grant permission for it to review outpatient services also, although none has yet begun to carry out such reviews. PSROs review the medical care provided, by utilization review of medical care for individuals and by medical care evaluation (MCE) studies. Utilization review can be either admission review, to determine the necessity for admission, or concurrent stay review, to determine the length of time a patient should be hospitalized. Under 1979 regulations, a system of concurrent review of elective surgical or major diagnostic or therapeutic procedures is required. If the PSRO believes that a procedure is being utilized inappropriately, the regulation requires that medical necessity review take place prior to the performance of the procedure (HCFA, 1979). In most instances, hospital committees are delegated by PSROs to perform these reviews, but PSROs must monitor the review process. Medical Care Evaluation studies are retrospective reviews of the medical care that was provided to certain groups of patients (e.g., by diagnosis), of the use of specific medical technologies, or of any category of medical or administrative services provided. As specified in the statute, PSROs review services to determine whether:

(A) such services and items are or were medically necessary;
(B) the quality of such services meets professionally recognized standards of health care; and
(C) in case such services and items are proposed to be provided in a hospital or other health care facility on an inpatient basis, such services and items could, consistent with the provision of appropriate medical care, be effectively provided on an outpatient basis or more economically in an inpatient health care facility of a different type.

The law requires that PSROs use norms, criteria, and standards in evaluating medical services. This approach allows nonphysicians to perform many of the reviews and also enhances the objectivity of the review process. Standards are developed by a consensus of physicians, based on typical patterns of practice in the area and on such regional or national information as may be available and considered applicable by the PSRO.

In its early stages, the PSRO program has concentrated on determining the need for hospitalization. Now PSROs are beginning to move beyond the question of necessity for hospitalization, to review of surgical procedures and review of ancillary services, including such radiological services as CT scanning.

PSRO decisions on medical care utilization and quality can be enforced in several ways. Reimbursement for services provided can be withheld by Medicare and Medicaid (Medicaid regulations are established in each state and vary somewhat). For serious and repeated violations of PSRO standards, a physician's right to be reimbursed through Medicare and Medicaid can be suspended or revoked.

The PSRO program is too new to evaluate definitively. Several evaluations have shown that PSRO reviews have led to a reduction in days of hospital care of Medicare enrollees. Whether the financial saving is large enough to offset the cost of the program has not been established. The overall effects of PSROs on quality of medical care are completely unknown (Congressional Budget Office, 1979; Office of Planning, Evaluation, and Legislation, 1977).

Shortcomings of the PSRO Program

Potential uses of many technologies are virtually unlimited. A principal issue, then, is how to ensure appropriate use. How can limits on use be established without sacrificing quality of care?

Historically, individual physicians have made decisions about appropriate use of a technology for each patient. Such decisions were based on clinical experience, advice from colleagues, information obtained from medical journals and manufacturers, judgment, and experience. As more physicians used a technology, usual and customary patterns of use developed. No formal process has existed for developing scientific information about the efficacy of medical technologies or for using that information as the basis for decisions about appropriate use.

The PSRO legislation established a framework by which appropriate use of medical technologies could be evaluated by physicians acting in organized groups rather than as individuals. Their decisions, however, are still based largely on traditional sources of information, so that customary practice patterns, whether appropriate or not, become accepted as standard. For most medical technologies, little is known about the four factors defining efficacy: benefits received and probability of benefit, population benefiting, medical problem affected, and appropriate conditions of care. Evaluating the overall efficacy of some technologies does pose problems. Nevertheless, the lack of scientifically derived information on indications for use hampers the development of appropriate standards. Provided with such information, PSROs could become a mechanism for evaluating medical care. In its absence, PSROs are developing local standards for medical services based primarily on prevailing patterns of medical practice.

The Health Standards and Quality Bureau (HSQB) does not have the authority to impose national standards for use. It does have the authority, but not the mandate, to collect the results of studies concerning efficacy and safety and to provide them to PSROs as model or recommended norms, criteria, and standards. Experience with the PSRO program seems to indicate that local PSROs have generally been willing to adopt, with minor modification, the model standards and criteria developed nationally. For example, draft criteria on computed tomography scanners, distributed in 1979, were being used by several PSROs by the end of that year (OTA, 1980).

Current Status of Quality Assurance

The programs described above have developed pragmatically as attempts to assure quality. However, their overall effectiveness and validity can easily be questioned.

The purpose of this section is to describe the state of the art of quality assessment and assurance. Partly this is to indicate the state of information that might be incorporated into existing assurance programs. But in a broader sense, it may give indications of what the future holds.

Research on the Quality of Medical Care

The research literature on assessing the quality of care is extensive, and a number of excellent bibliographies have been published (Brook, 1973; Donabedian, 1969, 1978a). A few important studies will be described here.

In 1953–54 a classic study of general practice in North Carolina used structure and process indicators. Taking the physicians' perspective, internists directly observed and rated the practitioners according to explicit criteria. The reviewers attached greatest importance to the process of diagnosis, and graded clinical performance according to the presence and use of certain technologies (Peterson et al., 1956). The study reported great variation in the level of professional performance.

Lembcke (1956) pioneered in developing the hospital medical audit, using analysis of clinical records. As an example, he evaluated major female pelvic surgery in several hospitals and found that the introduction of auditing techniques reduced both the population hysterectomy rate and the proportion of unnecessary hysterectomies.

During the 1950s and 1960s, Shapiro and his coworkers (1960, 1967,

1971) conducted a number of studies that examined the health outcomes of patients in a prepaid group practice. Perhaps the most noteworthy for medical technology was a comparison of mortality rates among the aged enrolled in the Health Insurance Plan of Greater New York (HIP) and the aged not so enrolled. The study found lower mortality rates for HIP enrollees in the eighteen months after the study year, a noteworthy result among an elderly group. HIP and non-HIP aged differed in their use of services: HIP patients were more likely to have received ancillary services and ambulatory services. However, a connection between different patterns of technology use and greater longevity was not established (Shapiro, 1967).

Trussel et al. (1962) studied the hospital care of members of the Teamsters Union and their families, in New York City, 1957–1961. The study used review of medical records, process and outcome techniques, and implicit criteria. The study found that only 57 percent of patients received "good or excellent medical care," while a fifth received poor care (1962, p. 25). A second study by this group in 1962, using similar evaluation techniques, arrived at similar conclusions (Morehead et al., 1964).

In the late 1960s and early 1970s a series of studies of the quality of medical care in Neighborhood Health Centers, primarily using process evaluation, showed that such auditing methods could be widely applied. As indicated by technology use in diagnoses, the quality of ambulatory care in Neighborhood Health Centers was found to be reasonably good when compared to other organized practice settings (Morehead, 1970; Morehead et al., 1971).

In the early 1970s, Kessner described a new approach to quality assessment called the Tracer Method. The approach had the advantage of examining both process and outcome, using a particular disease as a tracer. A tracer is a disease process with the following characteristics (Kessner et al., 1973, pp. 15–17):

1. A tracer should have a definite functional impact . . .
2. A tracer should be relatively well defined and easy to diagnose . . .
3. Prevalence rates should be high enough to permit the collection of adequate data from a limited population sample . . .
4. The natural history of the condition should vary with utilization and effectiveness of medical care . . .
5. The techniques of medical management of the condition should be well defined for at least one of the following processes: prevention, diagnosis, treatment or rehabilitation . . .
6. The effects of nonmedical factors on the tracer should be understood . . .

The tracer method has been applied to two different pediatric population groups in Washington, D.C. (Kessner and Kalk, 1973, pp. 15–17). Inappropriate or ineffective treatment was documented in a large proportion of the children.

Williamson (1978) has developed a method of quality assurance using medical conditions similar to tracers, based on health outcomes. Called health accounting, it involves providers in the assessment of their own work. The providers predict their outcomes in advance, and discrepancies between predictions and actual outcomes require action on their part. Although this method cannot be applied in many medical care settings, it has particular promise in organized ambulatory care situations.

Brook has pioneered in methods combining process and outcome measures (Brook, 1973; Brook and Appel, 1973). Brook and Appel (p. 1323) summarized their work as follows:

> To evaluate the procedures used to assess quality of care, five peer-review methods were compared. These methods involved judgments based on two kinds of data: what physicians did for the patients (process); and what happened to the patients (outcome). Criteria used to make judgments were either predetermined by group consensus (explicit), or selected subjectively by individual reviewers (implicit). The care of 296 patients with urinary-tract infection, hypertension or ulcerated gastric or duodenal lesions was reviewed with use of the five methods. Depending on the method, from 1.4 to 63.2 per cent of patients were judged to have received adequate care. Judgment of process using explicit criteria yielded the fewest acceptable cases (1.4 per cent). The largest differences found were between methods using different sources of data. Thus, medical care, judged with implicit criteria, was rated adequate for 23.3 per cent of patients with process, and 63.2 per cent when outcome was used.

Brook concluded that, although serious problems of method in assessing quality remain to be settled, as many as 25 per cent of patients would have had better outcomes if the medical processes had been better. Brook took a very optimistic position on the future of quality assurance activities of this type.

Rutstein et al. (1976) described an epidemiological (population-based) approach to quality evaluation. The approach counts cases of unnecessary disease and disability and unnecessary untimely deaths. The conditions used for the method were selected because critical increases in disease, disability, or death could serve as indexes of medical care quality. The approach uses an outcome technique to look at discrete instances of patient care. If an unnecessary event occurs, the circumstances surrounding the unnecessary event can be examined in detail. Brook has also pioneered in the use of outcome data (Avery et al., 1976; Brook et al., 1977).

Donabedian (1978b) has recently published an extensive discussion of past research in the area of quality assessment and assurance, including an extensive bibliography, in which he summarizes the state of the art. He states that an important reason for expanded quality assurance activities is " . . . the development, piece by piece, of the conceptual apparatus, the methods, and the technology of quality assessment and monitoring and their incorporation in several prototypes in actual practice."

This review of quality assessment and assurance activities shows the early stage of development of the field. In terms of technology, the standards set in quality assurance have little known relation to the efficacy of a particular intervention. Both structural and process standards are assumed to be related to favorable outcomes, but there is little tested validity to the assumptions. Indeed, a number of observers have said that the lack of generally accepted valid measures of quality remains one of the greatest problems in quality assessment and assurance activities (Donabedian, 1978a; Brook, 1973). It seems clear that much more evaluation of medical technology is a necessary precondition to effective quality assurance activities. It also seems clear that new organizational forms will be needed to establish the criteria for assessment, gather information on quality, disseminate the results of assessments, and take corrective action (Institute of Medicine, 1976). Cost implications and other social effects will also have to be incorporated. That remains the challenge for the future.

10
Selected Experience of Other Countries

> Refusal to accept the inevitable shortcomings of any society is responsible for a good deal of what is best in political life.
>
> Peter F. Drucker

The rise in the cost of medical care that has stimulated the questioning of medical technology in the United States has been paralleled in other countries. Virtually all industrialized countries have experienced rapid cost rises in the past few years. For example, costs rose 18.3 percent annually from 1970 to 1975 in the Netherlands; 21.5 percent annually in Australia for the same period; and 17.9 percent annually in Germany. These rapid rises have stimulated questions about the benefits of medical technology, very similar to those that have developed in the United States.

Other countries have policy mechanisms to deal with various stages of medical technology development and use that are similar to those of the United States. Questions about medical technology have led to attempts to use these mechanisms to channel or control medical technology.

Because of this common international concern, and because the scientific literature of this subject is very scanty, the Office of Technology Assessment commissioned a set of papers describing certain aspects of the health systems of a number of countries, including Canada, West Germany, France, the Netherlands, the United Kingdom, Sweden, Iceland, Japan, and Australia. The material in this chapter is drawn from those papers.[1]

In addition to a brief description of the country, its government and economy, and its health care system, each paper describes public policy mechanisms for dealing with each stage of medical technology development, diffusion, and use. In addition, authors of the papers were asked to

---
[1] Published by OTA in the summer of 1980.

provide information on how specific technologies were developed and diffused, and on policy mechanisms dealing with those technologies. This chapter will include materials on three of those technologies: computed tomography (CT) scanners, renal dialysis, and coronary bypass surgery.

Research and Development

As discussed in Chapter 3, medical technologies are the result of a complex process of research and development. As in the United States, other industrialized countries have assumed a major responsibility for the support of biomedical research and development of medical technology through governmental programs. Overall, the United States is the largest supporter of all R&D, accounting for 35 percent of the world's investment. Western European countries together account for about 22 percent of the world's total, and Eastern Europe and the USSR account for about 31 percent of the world's total (Annerstedt, 1979). Investments in health-related R&D make up about 7-10 percent of the total for all types of R&D.

Central government agencies in other countries carry out and support biomedical R&D, but probably no other country has one institution as dominant as the National Institutes of Health in the United States. In West Germany, for example, four Federal ministries support biomedical R&D— the Ministry for Research and Technology; the Ministry of Labor and Social Affairs; the Ministry for Youth, Family Affairs and Health; and the Ministry for Education and Science (Dumbaugh, 1979). Most of the Federally funded research is carried out through quasi-autonomous research institutes, such as the Max Planck Gesellschaft and the Deutsche Forschungsgesellschaft. However, much research is also carried out in universities and teaching hospitals, which are funded by the State governments. The Federal investment in biomedical R&D through these ministries is rather small, only about 97 million DM ($53 million) in 1978. That may be compared with 1.12 billion DM ($615 million) spent by the 25 leading German pharmaceutical companies on drug R&D in 1976.

In France, in contrast, the Central government is much more dominant (Fuhrer, 1979). Three public institutions support most of the biomedical R&D—The National Institute of Health and Medical Research, the National Center for Scientific Research, and the Universities. The two agencies do research, and also give grants and contracts. All scientific research is coordinated by an Under Secretary for Research attached to the Prime Minister's office. In 1978, France invested 1,400 million francs ($329 million) of public funds in biomedical R&D.

How these programs set priorities has not been well described (Rettig et al., 1974). Klein (1976) commented that biomedical research priorities in Britain have tended to be shaped by the interests of the research community rather than by an appraisal of what type of research would yield the greatest dividend to the community at large. However, there are signs of change. In Germany, for example, the stated objective of the Ministry of Research and Technology is to develop medical technology that would improve patient care, reduce side effects, and be more cost effective (Dumbaugh, 1979).

Evaluation of Medical Technology

In Chapters 6, 7, and 8, different forms of evaluation of medical technology and their use in the United States were described. The evaluation of efficacy and safety was emphasized as a particularly important function for government support.

Apparently, the level of evaluation activity in other countries is generally even lower than it is in the United States. Sweden has supported some clinical trials and other evaluations of medical technologies (Jonsson and Marke, 1977; Neuhauser and Jonsson, 1974; Gaensler et al., 1979). England has carried out a number of well-known controlled clinical trials oriented to efficacy and safety, primarily through the government-funded Medical Research Council (Stocking, 1979; Cochrane, 1972). In France, a small number of clinical trials have been funded by Central government agencies. In recent years, the French government has begun to fund cost-effectiveness studies (Fuhrer, 1979; Blanpain and Deleise, 1976, pp. 190–210).

Although the amounts devoted to such evaluations are small, a great deal of discussion goes on concerning expanding such activities. An international workshop in Stockholm, in September 1979, discussed the importance of doing more studies and also of collaborating internationally (Spri, 1979). Participants in the conference stated that they rely on the United States very heavily to evaluate new medical technologies, but are increasingly recognizing the need to do more studies themselves. They also proposed that such international organizations as the European Common Market and the World Health Organization should become involved and perhaps even coordinate international studies. An international European study of coronary bypass surgery in the mid-1970s was put forward as an example of cooperative effort (Neuhauser and Jonsson, 1974), and there were discussions during 1979 about a Common-Market-supported study of electronic fetal monitoring.

There are also some indications of increasing activity within countries. Australia now allocates about $1.5 million a year, through the Federal Department of Health, to health services research, including evaluations of such technologies as coronary care units and renal dialysis (Sax, 1979). In Germany, the Federal Ministry for Research and Technology is planning to begin evaluations of new diagnostic tests, laboratory equipment, and radiotherapy. As in the United States, evaluations tend to focus on drugs and medical equipment. In Germany, there is some concern about excessive surgery and thus it is being proposed that more evaluation is needed (Dumbaugh, 1979).

In contrast to the lack of formal experimental evaluations of medical technology, activities to synthesize existing knowledge are common. As Klein (1976) notes in England, physician consensus often substitutes for either scientific evaluation or public involvement. The same has been noted for Sweden (Blanpain and Deleise, 1976, p. 46; Gaensler et al., 1979). In Australia, the establishment of an expert national advisory panel on applications and costs of modern technology was recommended in a 1978 report, and will probably take place. The panel would advise on whether a new technology is of broad use or for specific types of patients, whether medical benefits should be paid for a new technology, whether benefits should be paid during further evaluation, and what impact the introduction of a new technology could be expected to have (Sax, 1979). In Canada, the provinces usually establish a joint Federal-Provincial committee or working party when new or expanded services are proposed (Needleman, 1979). For example, in 1975 the Working Party on Special Care Units in Hospitals published guidelines covering nine units or programs—including renal dialysis, cardiac care, nuclear medicine, intensive care, and narcotic addiction treatment.

Regulation of the Safety and Efficacy of Drugs and Medical Devices

As noted in Chapter 6, drugs and devices must be determined to be safe and efficacious, as defined by legislation, before they can be marketed in the United States.

Most countries have controls over drugs similar to those of the United States. However, direct regulation is generally not so stringent, although the trend is in that direction. Thus, in 1978 West Germany began to implement a program for drug regulation modelled after the U.S. Food and

Drug Administration (FDA). The Netherlands government runs a commission on drugs that advises the Minister of Health—without approval, a drug cannot be marketed in the Netherlands (Groot, 1979). Drug composition, efficacy, and safety are scrutinized by this commission. In Canada, the United Kingdom, and Japan, regulation is done similarly (Needleman, 1979; Broida, 1979).

In other countries, however, indirect controls over drugs are more important. For example, in France, drugs must meet certain standards of efficacy and safety to be marketed. But France also exercises indirect control through its decisions on whether a specific drug will be placed on the reimbursable formulary of the Social Security System. To be placed on this list, new drugs must be either more efficacious, have fewer side effects, and/or cost less than present formulary drugs (Fuhrer, 1979).

A recent agreement has provided that, if a drug as been approved for marketing in any two European Economics Commission countries, then the other countries will grant permission easily.

The 1976 medical devices legislation in the United States provides for device regulation. Other countries do not usually directly regulate medical equipment. Nonetheless, evaluation of medical devices is common, especially of their technical capabilities. In England, evaluation of a particular piece of equipment may be suggested by the National Health Service, by an individual researcher, or by a committee of the Medical Research Council. The Medical Research Council is responsible for most clinical trials (Stocking, 1979). In France, devices are not regulated, but they must be assessed as efficacious by the Social Security System to be reimbursed (Fuhrer, 1979). A certain amount of evaluation of devices is carried out in Germany by the Ministry of Research and Technology, and regulation of devices is being discussed (Dumbaugh, 1979). In Japan, devices are regulated for quality and efficacy by the Ministry of Health and Welfare (Broida, 1979).

Regulation: Health Planning

Chapter 4 also described the health planning law and its provision for certificate-of-need control over capital investment. Such an approach is common in other countries.

In France, for example, the Central government regulates the availability of certain resources for geographic areas and population groups (Fuhrer, 1979). For facilities and equipment that are best assessed from a national perspective, interregional planning and decisionmaking is done centrally with the assistance of the National Commission on Medical Equipment. The Ministry has a list of "heavy equipment" that require approval for acquisition. In 1979, there were eleven technologies on the heavy equipment list, including CT scanners, autoanalyzers, heart-lung machines, linear accelerators, and artificial kidneys. This mechanism can affect the capital expenditures of an institution and determine the availability of specialty units, beds, and personnel.

In Canada, the planning process is similar to that in France, but is decentralized to the provincial government level. The usual course of events is that a request from a provider for a new technology triggers a process of developing standards and criteria, and results in a provincial plan (Needleman, 1979). These plans have different degrees of force in different provinces. In Quebec, for example, the scope of provincial authority has been great since 1976, when regional councils were given considerable authority over the expenditure of substantial funds. In that province, the regional councils have been active in consolidating services to achieve economies.

In Britian, most purchases are controlled at the regional level, with very tight budget constraints (Stocking, 1979). However, certain pieces of equipment, such as x-ray apparatus, renal dialysis machines, and automated laboratory equipment, are purchased on centrally negotiated contracts. Even in most of these cases, the regional authorities may decide not to invest in a particular kind of equipment. Only in a few instances, such as for x-ray and radiotherapy equipment, are orders actually placed by the central government. Each regional authority tends to have an equipment budget, and there are committees at the regional level to decide on equipment purchases.

In Australia, there are essentially no controls on the investments of private hospitals (Sax, 1979). Public hospitals, however, must turn to state governments for capital expenditures above $50,000. State governments usually make such decisions with the assistance of expert committees. There are attempts to regionalize the hospital system in Australia and to control technology more stringently.

In Germany, planning for hospital services is a function of the states, but a 1972 Federal law on capital investments in hospitals requires a regionalized hospital system (Dumbaugh, 1979). Under this law, bed needs are planned by the states, and there is the beginning of a trend toward centralization of highly sophisticated technology.

In Japan, there is apparently no control over capital investment or the purchase of machines (Broida, 1979).

Controls on the Use of Technology

This section will discuss the last several items from the outline presented in the beginning of the chapter: utilization review, financing, and using the results of evaluation. The use of technology can be directly regulated—as when it is illegal to use a technology—or indirectly regulated—as when the insurance mechanism will not pay for use of the technology. In the United States, as described in Chapter 5, the reimbursement system has seldom been used purposely to influence the use of technologies. On the other hand, since passage of the 1972 legislation establishing the PSRO program (Chapter 9), hospital services provided under the Medicare and Medicaid program have been more directly regulated.

In other countries, direct regulation controls are limited. In Germany, only rudimentary comparisons of utilization can be done (Dumbaugh, 1979). Utilization controls in Canada focus on outpatient care and are designed to identify fraud or high-billing physicians (Needleman, 1979).

The fee mechanism, in countries that use fee-for-service as the method of reimbursement, is used only infrequently to directly influence utilization, although it does of course have an effect in those instances. In France, more complex technological procedures are associated with a higher rate of reimbursement, so the incentive is to perform more complex procedures, just as it is in the United States (Fuhrer, 1979). In Japan, new technologies are readily added to the fee schedule (Broida, 1979). In Australia, the fee schedule encourages the rapid and uncontrolled diffusion of new technology (Sax, 1979). In Germany, fee schedules are not used consciously to affect utilization of technology (Dumbaugh, 1979). In the Netherlands, the fees encourage the expansion of technology (Groot, 1979).

However, in Australia, there have been discussions about using fee schedules as an effective cost-containment device. So far, physicians have prevented use of schedules in this way (Sax, 1979). In Canada, fee schedules are being used somewhat to change incentives. For example, the physician fees for renal dialysis have been reduced in Ontario (Needleman, 1979). In the Netherlands, the radiologists recently made a new fee agreement, whereby their fees would be decreased by a percentage above a certain number of examinations—presumably, this decreases the incentive to do extra tests (Groot, 1979).

A few mechanisms deserve further comment. Budget constraints seem likely to be an effective method for controlling both technology and medical care costs. Therefore, the global hospital budget system of Canada and the prospective budgets of the United Kingdom will be described below. In Sweden, medical services are funded at the county level, which leads the population of each county to be concerned about the services that are being offered and their costs.

In Canada, the hospital budgeting system is the central process by which resource allocation decisions are made (Needleman, 1979). The process has two parts: the establishment of the operating budget for the hospital, and the capital budget. In Ontario, the province generally provides two-thirds of the capital funds for an approved construction or renovation. Hospitals may fund a project totally from a hospital's capital funds, providing that the program will not cause additional operating costs. Over the last several years, only limited capital funds have been provided to the hospitals in Ontario. In addition to limitations on construction funds, certain services must be approved by the province. These include diagnostic radiology, therapeutic radiology, nuclear medicine, data processing, laboratory automation, and anesthesia and recovery equipment. This approach has been successful in containing costs. Since 1975, as the percentage of the GNP devoted to health care has risen in the United States, that of Canada has stayed about the same, 7.2 percent (Hatcher, 1979). The effects of this constraint on technology, on the health of the population, or on other factors have not been documented.

In the United Kingdom, budgeting for the National Health Service is done centrally and allocated to regions on the basis of a complex formula that includes population and various factors, such as standardized mortality ratios, that might indicate the need for health care (Stocking, 1979). The philosophy of the system is that the upper levels provide a coordinating and policy-making function, while actual management of health services occurs at lower levels. Each region must operate on the basis of a limited budget, and this has been quite effective in restraining cost rises. In 1978, health services expenditure was about 5.7 percent of GNP. As indicated in earlier sections, most decisions concerning technology are in fact made at the local level within these budget constraints. Capital budgets are developed and allocated to regions in a way similar to that for revenue costs. With a fairly conservative attitude in Britain toward technology, pressures do not develop for acquiring new technology to the same extent that they do in the United States (see tables 10–1, 10–2, and 10–3.) Nonetheless, some people feel that technology gets priority funding over less glamorous services, such as care of the elderly and handicapped. These decisions, which are made at the regional and local level, are obviously political, and specialists are often able to argue successfully for the necessity of a particular technology.

In Sweden, services are regionalized, with a hierarchical organization of services with a regional, specialized hospital at the top (Gaensler et al., 1979). This hierarchical system aims to prevent unnecessary duplication of technology-intensive specialities. (Many of the aspects of services within each region also apply to the organization of services in Iceland—see Gunnarson and Neuhauser, 1979.) As a result, neurology, radiation therapy, thoracic surgery, neurosurgery, pediatric surgery, and certain types of cardiac care are provided only through the regional hospital. However, the system also allows provision of services at the most cost-effective level (intuitively defined), which often is the health center. Physicians and health centers, as well as district hospitals, are controlled at the county level and funded by the county. The fact that Swedes pay the highest taxes in the developed world, including heavy taxes to cover medical care, testifies to their desires for access to the best medical care. Sweden has not contained the rising costs of medical care, and its health care expenditures were about 9 percent of GNP in 1978, similar to that of the United States. But the regionalized system may have prevented waste and duplication, at least in the cases of the CT scanner and cardiac surgery (see below).

Specific Technologies

The purpose of this section is to indicate what the effect of some of these policies and programs may have been on the diffusion and use of selected medical technologies. The technologies presented are expensive and visible. They are not necessarily the major technological contributors to rising costs, nor are they representative of all medical technology. In fact, most medical technology is inexpensive individually, as in the case of clinical laboratory services, and only expensive in the aggregate. These cases have been chosen for one reason: data are available on them and specific policies have often dealt with them. It is worth stressing that the implications of these data for the health of the population, use of other technologies, and so forth, have not been demonstrated. The data are presented because they are interesting and because they indicate the need for further research.

Computed Tomography (CT) Scanner

The CT scanner is a revolutionary diagnostic device that combines x-ray equipment with a computer and a cathode ray tube to produce images of cross sections of the human body. Machines are available that scan the head; another type can scan any part of the body, including the head. CT scanning was developed in Britain in the late 1960s, and was quickly hailed as the greatest advance in radiology since the discovery of x-rays. The 1979 awarding of a Nobel prize to the inventors has made it official. CT scanning has been rapidly and enthusiastically accepted by the medical community. Since the average cost of each machine is more than $500,000, their rapid spread has caused most countries to become involved in the planning of the location of scanners.

Controls over scanners have ranged over almost all possibilities. In Japan and Iceland, there have been no controls (Broida, 1979; Gunnarson and Neuhauser, 1979). In Sweden, decisions are made at the county level, but information on CT scanners was developed by a central research unit (which was partially funded by county councils) and this unit has influenced decisionmaking (Gaensler et al., 1979). In Australia, purchase of CT scanners by public hospitals is controlled by each state, and the states are presently opposed to additional scanners (Sax, 1979). In the United Kingdom and in Canada, decisions are made at the regional and provincial level within budget constraints (Stocking, 1979; Needleman, 1979). In the U.K., however, the national Department of Health and Social Security recommended that each region purchase at least one head scanner. In Ontario, Canada, the province has set a guideline of one scanner per 500,000 population. In Germany, scanners are financed by the central government after an application for procurement has passed through the state (Dumbaugh, 1979). In the Netherlands, the government has no relevant authority, but hospitals agreed not to install a scanner without government approval. The government has set a guideline of one head scanner per 500,000 population (Groot, 1979). Finally, in France, scanner purchases are regulated centrally under a guideline of one scanner (either head or body) per million population (Fuhrer, 1979).

Table 10–1 shows the number of scanners in each of these countries. The table shows that some countries have been successful in restricting the diffusion of CT scanners. However, the one country without any CT scanner, Iceland, has had no restrictions on purchase. This should raise cautions about trying to read too much into the reasons behind the data. Another interesting aspect of the table is that most countries have focused on purchasing head scanners, which are less expensive. Many would consider that the body scanner has not established itself as an essential part of the diagnostic armamentarium.

Direct controls on technology in physicians' offices are not common. In most countries, a degree of skepticism about medical technology and the large investments required prevent expensive technologies from being diffused into nonhospital settings. In some countries, such as Britain, office practice has traditionally included only limited access to sophisticated medical technology. However, in the United States, about 18 percent of CT scanners are in nonhospital settings, and in Germany, 30 percent of CT scanners are in physicians' offices.

Table 10-1.
Number of Installed CT Scanners, by Country, 1978 and 1979

Country	March 1978				1979			
	Head	Body	Total	Per million population	Head	Body	Total	Per million population
United States	337	668	1005	4.6	400	854	1254	5.7 (Feb.)
Japan	180	112	292	2.6	304	212	516	4.6 (Apr.)
Netherlands	U	U	U	U	U	U	39	2.8 (Dec.)
West Germany	51	42	93	1.5	U	U	160	2.6 (Jul.)
Australia	U	U	U	U	7	21	28	1.9 (Jan.)
Sweden	8	5	13	1.6	8	6	14	1.7 (Jan.)
Canada	U	U	U	U	9	29	38	1.7 (May)
United Kingdom	36	16	52	0.9	39	18	57	1.0 (Jan.)
France	10	2	12	0.2	20	10	30	0.6 (Jan.)
Iceland	0	0	0	0.0	0	0	0	0.0 (Sep.)

Note: In France, an additional 21 scanners were authorized in July 1979. Iceland plans to buy at least one scanner.
Key to Symbols: U = Unknown
Sources: OTA Country Papers; Jonsson (1978). Canadian data were furnished to OTA by the Government of Canada, Ottawa.

Finally, government regulations do not always have the intended effects, and this again raises cautions about concluding that government policies are responsible for the distribution of technology. In Ontario, Canada, the province has approved seven CT scanners, but three unauthorized scanners are also functioning in Toronto (Needleman, 1979). The government has applied no sanctions against these hospitals. In France, a restrictive policy on imports was developed to allow the French company, CGR, to develop a scanner for the domestic market (Fuhrer, 1979). The restrictive policies led to 15 scanners' being purchased without government subsidies, and most of these are in private establishments. In the U.K., the government attempted to slow the diffusion of body scanners, and thereby caused hospitals to buy scanners without government support, either through endowment funds or from funds raised by appeals or by private donors (Stocking, 1979).

Renal Dialysis

Renal dialysis is the process of removing toxic waste products from the blood by means of an artificial kidney. Since about 1960, long-term dialysis has been possible. For patients with end-stage renal disease, the alternative to long-term dialysis is often death. Another intervention that is often successful and is considerably cheaper is transplantation. Renal transplantation is a surgical procedure whereby a healthy kidney from some other human or a kidney from a recently dead person (cadaver) is substituted for an individual's nonfunctioning kidney. The problem with transplantation is that the body tends to reject a kidney from another person.

Generally speaking, the countries discussed in this paper have fully covered dialysis for people with end-stage renal disease, through their health insurance programs, since the 1960s. Since the rate of end-stage renal disease is similar in developed countries, and those with end-stage renal disease will die without treatment, one might expect to find similar rates of dialysis from country to country. Such is not the case.

Table 10–2 summarizes available data on dialysis in each country. First, it is notable that numbers of new patients entering end-stage renal disease programs vary by a factor of at least two. One reason this could be true is that it was not the policy in the Netherlands, for example, to dialyze those under the age of 15, and those over 60 were quite often not dialyzed, although that policy is changing (Groot, 1979). In the U.K., also, those over the age of 60 often are not dialyzed (Stocking, 1979). In the U.K., Stocking attributes the difference primarily to conservatism among clini-

Table 10-2.
Treatment of Patients with End-Stage Renal Disease, per Million Population, by Country and Year

Country	New Patients 1976	Patients on Dialysis or with a Functioning Transplant		Transplant Rates 1976
		1975	1978	
United States	U	U	164[1,2]	15.9
Netherlands	21.4	90	U	11.7
Sweden	28.7	85	73[1]	20.0
United Kingdom	15.1	62	92	10.8
West Germany	30.8	88	114	U
France	29.1	102	133[1] (1977)	6.8
Canada	31.4	121.1 (1976)	U	15.1
Australia	U	U	77[1]	U
Iceland	U	42	U	U
Japan	U	140 (1976)	222	U

Key to Symbols: U = Unknown
[1] = Dialysis only
[2] = Approximate figure

Sources: OTA Country Papers; Office of Health Economics; Department of Health and Human Services (personal communication). Canadian data furnished by the Government of Canada, Ottawa.

cians, since unused dialysis places have been available. However, this has since become a national issue in Britain: new places are being developed, and the rate of new patients has risen from 15.1 per million in 1976 to 19.0 per million in 1978. This factor, plus the additional people entering the program each year, leads to ever-growing numbers and expense.

The choice of dialysis or transplant is also interesting. Based on the limited data available, it appears that the Netherlands depends on dialysis and does relatively fewer transplants. It is worth noting that the Netherlands government has tried to increase the number of transplants, but has been unsuccessful because of a limited number of kidneys (Groot, 1979). Sweden, on the other hand, relies more on transplants.

Another policy issue is the setting of dialysis. Dialysis in the home is recognized as being more economically efficient, yet home dialysis is not very common in the United States, France, or Japan. In Germany, 30 percent of dialysis is done at home. In the United States, the figure is about 25 percent (Rettig, 1979b). In the U.K., about two-thirds of those being dialyzed are on home dialysis (Stocking, 1979). It seems likely that budget constraints on the regions have led to this more economical form of dialysis.

Coronary Bypass Surgery

Coronary bypass surgery is a surgical procedure in which a graft is put on a blocked or partially blocked coronary artery to bypass the constricted portion of the artery. Coronary bypass surgery is controversial because it was rapidly accepted in the United States without adequate clinical trials to demonstrate its efficacy. As evidence has accumulated, it appears that coronary bypass surgery does extend life of those with narrowing of the left main coronary artery. That condition occurs in about 10 to 15 percent of those with severe coronary artery disease. In addition, advocates argue that the surgery is an effective and appropriate therapy to relieve the pain of angina pectoris.

The countries discussed in this paper do fewer coronary bypass procedures per capita than are done in the United States (Table 10–3). Although the table gives data only for certain years, it is clear that the United States rate is considerably above that of other countries. If the number of operations performed in 1979 in the United States reached the 100,000 figure predicted by some, the rate would then be almost 450 per million.

In this case, a combination of physician skepticism and lack of facilities for open heart surgery have limited the procedure in other countries. In the U.K., Sweden, Australia, France, and the Netherlands, there are limitations on the number of units that can do such surgery (Stocking, 1979; Fuhrer, 1979; Gaensler et al., 1979; Sax, 1979; Groot, 1979). In

Table 10–3.
Coronary Artery Surgery per Million Population, by Country and Year

Country	1975	1977	1978
United States	280	369	U
Canada	129	160 (1976)	U
Netherlands	50	U	325[3]
Sweden	24	20	U
United Kingdom	25	55[1]	U
West Germany	14	20[4]	U
France	U	U	19
Australia	U	136	U
Iceland	U	U	233[2]

Key to Symbols: U = Unknown
    [1] = England and Wales only
    [2] = All sent abroad, figure is estimated
    [3] = An estimated 3500 procedures done in the Netherlands, plus 1000 abroad.
    [4] = Approximate figures
Sources: OTA Country Papers; National Center for Health Statistics; Government of Canada, personal communication; World Health Organization (1978); and Preston (1977), p. 173.

Germany, there are no restrictions, but seven large centers do most of the open heart surgery in the country (Dumbaugh, 1979). In Iceland, such open heart surgery is not performed. In addition, physicians have been overtly skeptical of the procedure in the U.K., Sweden, and France (Stocking, 1979; Gaensler et al., 1979; Fuhrer, 1979).

In Iceland and the Netherlands, the patient demand for the procedure has led those countries to pay for patients to go to other countries for coronary bypass (Gunnarson and Neuhauser, 1979; Groot, 1979). There are waiting lists in the Netherlands and Germany, and political pressures to increase the available facilities.

Gaensler et al. (1979) have used this case to discuss issues involved in finding the best route to reaching optimal use of a technology:

> The pattern in the U.S. seems to be over-expansion followed by contraction. The disadvantage of this path is that resources are wasted. Furthermore, reducing the share of resources allocated to an entrenched (technology) is more difficult than expanding it. Sweden's 'wait and see' approach was cost-effective but had one major drawback. During the 'trial' period . . . many deserving candidates were not given treatment or put on waiting lists.

That indeed is the dilemma of attempting to manage technology.

Discussion

The countries discussed in this paper have begun to be concerned about the costs and benefits of medical technology. Their more coherent systems already have made it possible for some of them to develop specific policies related to medical technology. It may be that many approaches used in other countries have applicability in the United States.

Russell has analyzed policies toward medical technology in some other developed countries, and has stated that policies toward medical technology can be organized into a hierarchy (1979, pp. 132–155). Each step of the hierarchy represents a growing commitment to cost containment over other goals. At the first level, the government may try to promote the adoption of new technologies. Most countries have done this by paying for new technologies (perhaps even paying more than for existing technologies) or by assuring that sufficient people are trained to provide the new technology. At the second level, the government may concern itself with whether the technologies are being used efficiently. Without asking questions about the benefits of the technology, the government may ask if more services could be produced for the same cost. They may concern themselves with duplication and access. These first two steps assume that technology is a good thing and leave judgments about benefits to the medical profession and to patients. Until recently, public policies toward technology have focused on these two levels. But, increasingly, there is concern that technologies have not been proved to be of value, or that certain technologies are being used inappropriately. The government can approach this question by relying on expert advice (panels, commissions), or it may begin to ask whether rigorous studies such as randomized clinical trials have proved the technology to be of benefit and acceptably safe. Although there has yet been little linkage in other countries between demands for rigorous proof and public policies that could control medical technology, it is being actively discussed and seems inevitable. Finally, at the fourth level, the government accepts the possibility that it may not be desirable to provide every kind of care that has some benefit, whatever the cost. The question then shifts from whether the technology is beneficial to whether it is beneficial *enough* (Fuchs, 1974).

The United States, too, is beginning to ask the question, "Is the technology beneficial enough?"

11
Strategies for Improvement

> If the trumpet give an uncertain sound, who shall prepare himself to the battle?
>
> Corinthians 14:8

Appropriate use of any technology requires consideration of efficacy, safety, costs, and social effects. Overuse of a technology may lead to both excessive expenditures and unwarranted risk to patients. Underuse may result in delayed detection or prolongation of medical problems. In either case, the result is basic policy problems related to the appropriate use of medical technologies.

This book has discussed many factors that affect the use of medical technology. One obvious factor is the desire of physicians to provide good care for their patients. Medical education predisposes physicians to liberal use of technologies by emphasizing thoroughness in diagnosis, rather than discrimination, and by encouraging excessive faith in the efficacy of therapeutic technologies. Fear of malpractice situations further encourages overuse of medical technology, especially diagnostic technologies such as laboratory tests. As third-party payment in its present form has increased,

> the benefit required to justify a decision in the eyes of doctors and patients has declined. This has led to increased use of resources in all sorts of ways—including the introduction of technologies that otherwise might not have been adopted at all and, more often, the more rapid and extensive diffusion of technologies that had already been adopted to some extent [Russell, 1978].

And finally, with imperfect information to indicate how best to help the patient, the physician is handicapped in decisionmaking.

Several Federal agencies develop information on the benefits, costs, and risks of medical technologies, but no public or private agency has yet established a formal, systematic process to develop and disseminate needed information about medical technologies. Without such information, physicians either test technologies empirically or rely on the advice of trusted colleagues. This informal system can both retard the spread of valuable technologies and promote the use of questionable ones.

Prevailing methods of financing medical care provide incentives for additional use of medical technologies, regardless of their marginal value. A regulatory framework dealing with medical technologies has developed, partly in response to this situation.

This chapter will discuss options for improving policies toward medical technology—with the ultimate aim of improving the use of medical technology. We recognize that there are formidable obstacles to improvement in the existing system. Existing value and belief systems, reward and incentive systems, and patterns of economic and political domination all support the present system. The societal emphasis on curative, technological medicine that has developed over the past decades has its own inertia (Mahler, 1975). It is expressed in the orientation of the NIH, with its emphasis on the traditional biomedical paradigm of Cartesian mechanism and its lack of emphasis on social science and epidemiology. It is expressed in the medical empires that have grown up around medical schools, with their concentrations of technology and specialists and their technologically oriented education for medical students and other future health care providers. It is expressed in the financing system that rewards medical and surgical procedures and does not encourage counseling and caring. It is expressed in profits for a large industry and hidden profits of major medical centers and providers. It is expressed in consumer demands for the latest in medical technology. And it is expressed in well-funded political lobbies and political action groups that fund political campaigns. We recognize these difficulties and are not sanguine that they will be faced rapidly. At the same time, the society has begun to question. The door is opening to change, not only in the United States, but in other countries as well. Consumer groups are fostering a new consciousness and developing tools to aid lay people in evaluating medical technology (Frost et al., 1979). We hope that we have revealed some of the biases behind possible choices. Thus, our purpose in this book was to analyze the problems associated with medical technology and to suggest leverage points that could be used to foster change. We hope that others will consider the political and social feasibility of these possibilities and use them in altering our existing societal mechanisms and agencies.

Options fall into six general classes: (1) Develop more effective guidance for biomedical research and development; (2) Change medical education to produce more discerning users of medical technology; (3) Examine the organization of medical practice; (4) Develop better information on efficacy, safety, costs, and social effects of medical technologies and disseminate it to users; (5) Strengthen regulatory programs; and (6) Use the financing system more aggressively to make the use of medical technologies more rational.

Controlling Biomedical Research and Technology Development

The costs of medical care and technology's contribution to those costs have led to proposals to control the process more effectively (Gaus, 1975). The Director of NIH has said, "A corollary problem is presented by palliative technologies, such as renal dialysis, applied at exorbitant cost in present-day clinical settings. The mounting demands that these be extended to every patient in need of them suggests that science has some obligation to anticipate the fruits of its research . . ." (Fredrickson, 1977). Indeed, the amount of contract money from NIH to support targeted research has consistently increased over the past few years (Frederickson, 1977).

We support the option of controlling biomedical research in only a limited way. As described in Chapter 3, basic research is impossible to plan in advance with any assurance of the result. Our view is that attempting to plan the results of such research would produce little improvement and has the potential for much harm. Furthermore, since Federal support for biomedical research is spread across a number of agencies, collecting information on these programs is difficult. Perhaps the most serious impediment is the large amount of private research and development. Attempting to prevent development of a technology by refusing to fund it with public money would have little effect if private industry (or the governments of other countries) decided to develop it. The decision would still have to be faced later whether or not to incorporate the technology into the medical care system. The CT scanner, which was refined and originally manufactured in Britain, is an excellent example.

On the other hand, technology assessment, or anticipating the social impacts of medical technologies, might be useful in selected instances. A study conducted by NIH on the totally implantable artificial heart examined many ramifications of such a development, and may have caused a relative shift toward heart assist devices. Such assessments, which are included in the mandate of the National Center for Health Care Technology, might assist targeted research decisions in some cases.

Finally, we do support additional funding for areas of research slighted under our present system. The Cartesian paradigm has fostered halfway technology, while starving research on nutrition, epidemiology of disease, social science, and so forth. We believe that chronic disease can be more effectively confronted with new knowledge from these nontraditional health disciplines. We also favor new and additional funding for the evaluation of medical technology, as discussed below.

Changing Medical Education

Because this book has not discussed medical education in any detail, this option is not developed at length. Nonetheless, physicians are largely responsible for technology use, and it is ultimately their behavior that must change. The current training of physicians emphasizes the use of the latest procedures and equipment both because the medical faculty is so specialized and because teaching hospitals are at the forefront technologically (Ebert, 1977). Medical training also stresses that physicians refine their diagnoses with extensive tests as a means of doing all they can for their patients.

Physicians could be trained more effectively in the scientific method and in the conduct and interpretation of clinical trials (Jonas, 1978). They could also be guided to use technologies with more discretion and could be exposed to the cost implications of their decisions through information about patient's hospital bills (Cooper and Gaus, 1979). Fostering primary care practitioners through legislative action and changes in medical training is also a promising approach (Institute of Medicine, 1978).

Examining the Organization of Medical Practice

The organizational structure of medical practice has received little attention in the context of the adoption and use of technologies and the costs of care (Willems, 1979b). Most medical technologies are provided through hospitals and, increasingly, through group practices as well. But rarely is the delivery of care integrated. Most commonly, separate practices and organizations, such as physicians' offices, diagnostic facilities, and hospitals, provide fragments of care to patients.

Organizational structure may be an influential as well as unappreciated aspect of the medical care system. Complex organizations contain subgroups of decisionmakers who have different perspectives, and these differences may temper ultimate decisions about the adoption and use of technologies. More complex organizations also contain a wider range of technologies and bear the costs of their purchase and use.

Hypotheses about the effect of organization on technology remain to be tested, but certainly merit examination. Governmental programs, both indirectly by favoring regionalization and sharing of technologies and directly by promoting Health Maintenance Organizations, are encouraging changes in the organization of medical practice. At a minimum, the implications of such changes should be assessed. Ideally, we might support certain types of organization that are shown to make more judicious decisions about the adoption and use of technologies and provide an alternative to increasing direct regulatory activities (Mechanic, 1978; Prahalad and Abernathy, 1974).

Developing Information on Efficacy, Safety, Costs, and Social Effects

Most decisions concerning the use of medical technology depend directly or indirectly on the assessment of efficacy and safety. Although more knowledge about efficacy and safety does not necessarily assure that one can define appropriate use, it is impossible to define such use without that information. Information on efficacy and safety is necessary to physicians and to all those who must make decisions about medical technology, including hospital administrators, government regulators, and public and private third-party payers.

In an era of limited resources, it may also be necessary to begin to develop information on costs or cost effectiveness. The applicability of this information to the level of the individual physician and patient is problematic. Some would argue that it is the role of physicians to do all they can for their patients, and the role of the overall society to make resource allocation decisions. Whatever the wisdom, however, resource allocation decisions are being made. Costs do matter; physicians and hospitals do not provide all technologies to everyone. Better information and more informed decisions could increase the benefits and reduce the harm to the population.

The development of information on efficacy, safety, costs, and social effects requires setting priorities. For the information to be valuable, the technology to be studied must be identified, the appropriate evaluations conducted, and the results synthesized in a form accessible to users. The synthesized information must also be disseminated to the individuals and organizations that need it. The use of such information by regulatory agencies and financing programs is described below.

Although simple to delineate on paper, the process of developing information is complex and difficult to implement. It is essential to remember that such a process already occurs informally at present. The short-term suggestion is to formalize the process and make it more scientific. It may also be hoped that more evaluative studies will be done so that their results will be available in the future to be synthesized and disseminated. Without the scientific studies, the other activities are of dubious value.

Many questions will need to be addressed if this process is to be implemented as proposed by the Office of Technology Assessment (1978a) and the Technology Health Management Task Force. For example, when should evaluations be undertaken? Since technologies change as they diffuse into use and often improve with use, should studies by done later in the life cycle of the technology? Or should the studies be begun as soon as the new technology can be identified, so that the results can affect further diffusion? And what kind of evaluation is appropriate to each stage of technology? Perhaps an evaluation of early clinical experience could guide further diffusion, while large controlled clinical trials could be organized after early use suggests that the technology has some benefit. And how does one differentiate with reliability and validity between a technology that is highly efficacious and does not need to be evaluated by a complex controlled clinical trial (such as pencillin might have been), and a technology of modest benefit that may nonetheless be worth widespread use in selected instances? (Coronary bypass surgery might be an example.)

These questions can only be addressed over time as a system develops. The essence of our argument is that such a system is needed. There is presently only a limited attempt to develop such a system. The Federal Government's identification of medical technologies to study occurs in an ad hoc manner, with few efforts to coordinate the selections with the informational needs of relevant governmental agencies and private groups. Only the Food and Drug Administration has complete information, much of which is proprietary, on certain classes of technologies. The new National Center for Health Care Technology has begun to develop a priority list of technologies needing study, but it is not clear how or whether the list will influence ongoing activities.

It would also be possible to go a step beyond synthesis and arrive at conclusions or judgments about the value, risks, and appropriate use of a particular technology. These judgments could be actively disseminated to users and to the public, along with the supporting information.

Providing syntheses would add to the information individuals and organizations have available to them for making decisions. This information might reduce errors in judgment that such individuals and organizations make under the present informal system. This assumes that credible syntheses are possible and that involving the most knowledgeable people in making judgments would usually lead to a better conclusion. We believe that both are true.

The development and dissemination of information to individual physicians is not controversial. Almost everyone agrees that, though perhaps costly, it could do no harm and would probably do quite a lot of good.

Information on the efficacy and safety of medical technologies seems to affect physician behavior. For example, the results of the University Group Diabetes Program (UGDP) trial of oral treatment for diabetes appears to have led to a marked reduction in prescribing of Orinase, the most commonly used oral therapy (Levy, 1980). A study of the most efficient diagnostic approach to renovascular hypertension seems to have had an effect on practice (McNeil, 1980). Little research has been done on the effects of such trials and, so, little information is available on methods of organizing effective dissemination activities. It seems likely, however, that definitive syntheses could have more effect than published clinical trials that have not been actively disseminated to practitioners.

Developing information for groups, especially Federal agencies, is more controversial. For example, judgments could be used to determine which technologies would be covered by financing programs (see later in this chapter). These judgments would then become the focus of considerable political and economic pressure.

Strengthening Regulatory Programs

Partially as an attempt to offset powerful incentives encouraging the use of medical technologies, Congress has established three regulatory programs: the FDA, the PSRO program, and the capital review (or planning) program. All of these programs have obvious weaknesses. Private physicians' offices are largely excluded from capital expenditure review despite their importance. And about 20 percent of CT scanners in the United States, representing a capital investment of more than $100 million, are operating in physicians' offices. After marketing approval, FDA does not have authority to restrict subsequent use of drugs and devices by patients or physicians.

However, we do not propose use of these regulatory programs as the main policy tool for managing health care technology, because we doubt their ultimate utility for this purpose. The FDA processes stem from the philosophy that "in a complex society, individual consumers can no longer protect their own interests and the government must therefore do it for them" (Hutt, 1976). The FDA gives a minimal degree of protection against unsafe or ineffective drugs and devices. It is a powerful mechanism for dealing with a relatively clear-cut case, and its power over marketing is sufficient for those cases. However, it does not influence utilization once a product is approved for marketing.

We are skeptical about the power of the PSRO program and the capital review program to have a great influence on utilization of technologies. It is obvious that the capital review and the PSRO programs often lack the best scientific information on which to make their decisions. Even if the results of randomized controlled clinical trials of a technology are available, that information alone will probably not answer the question of interest to health planners: How many scanners should we allow in this area? Likewise, available studies will only partially answer the questions asked by PSROs: What is appropriate use of this technology, and what acceptable standards of use should be defined? The new National Center for Health Care Technology was created in part to meet this need. Only time will tell whether it is successful in meeting some rather formidable challenges.

As noted earlier, these programs have been developed partly as an attempt to deal with financial and other incentives that promote the rapid, and often premature, application of technology. However, the literature on regulation leads one to predict that the programs will not be able to achieve their goals. As noted by Enthoven and Noll (1979):

> If a regulator attempts to make the regulated behave in a way that is directly opposed to their financial interests, regulated entities will have a strong incentive to attempt to bend, fight, or evade regulations. This will force regulators to deal with many individual cases and will subject them to continuing pressure to grant exceptions to their general policies.

It is certainly clear that regulation through the PSRO program and other programs have failed both to control rising costs of hospital care and to develop and maintain satisfactory standards of quality (Noll, 1975; Congressional Budget Office, 1979). Likewise, the capital review program has not had notable effects. For example, it seems to have had little effect on the diffusion of CT scanners, the major test for such agencies in the last five years (OTA, 1980).

There is growing interest in using incentives to achieve the goals of regulatory programs (Enthoven and Noll, 1979; Schultze, 1977). Moreover, changing the reimbursement system could help make regulation more effective, if the financial incentives toward rapid acceptance of medical technology were eased.

Financing the Use of Medical Technologies

The climate of public policy has changed greatly since language in the 1965 legislation establishing Medicare warned the program not to interfere with the practice of medicine. Experience since that time has indicated that third-party payment by its very existence affects medical practice and the use of technologies (Iglehart, 1977). The recent groundswell of proposals for changing financing arrangements reflects the acceptance of that fact. If one assumes that financing affects technology use, failure to be attentive to the implications of the arrangements could result in missed opportunities to guide use in socially desirable directions, and is tacit acceptance of whatever patterns of use develop (Institute of Medicine, 1978).

Attention to financing has other reasons to commend it. Theoretically, each use of medical resources competes with alternative uses. This competition is fairly visible and overt within governmental agencies, such as HHS and the VA. Greater expenditure on the provision of currently covered services reduces the funding available for categorial programs, such as health promotion or access improvement, and for the expansion of coverage into new areas such as disease prevention (Mechanic, 1978).

Moreover, financing arrangements represent an indirect approach to influence technology use. Incentives are more congenial to American social and political values. In contrast to regulation, which seeks directly to accomplish an effect, the leverage of financing may indirectly channel use through the incentives created. The strength of that leverage depends on the importance of third-party payment to hospitals, physicians, and patients.

Present third-party payment covers, and therefore encourages, excessive reliance on technology by patients, physicians, and hospitals. As a result, technologies are often used when they have little effect, provide only duplicative information, or add unnecessary costs.

An option that has gained increasing acceptance since the advent of CT scanning is making third-party payment conditional on an evaluation of a technology's efficacy and safety. This policy seeks to avoid payment for the use of technology that is inefficacious compared to alternatives. Medicare, under the section of its legislation limiting payment to services that are reasonable and necessary, has evaluated and, on occasion, denied payment for certain technologies. Since the case of CT scanning, these reviews have gone beyond clearly outmoded technologies to those more controversial. The evaluation procedure is also becoming more systematic.

In the private sector, Blue Cross/Blue Shield has taken similar steps. The national organization recommended that local plans establish appropriate indications for CT body scans. Under its Medical Necessity Program, the organization will pay for certain outmoded or inefficacious procedures only if physicians justify their use.

While less intrusive than directly prohibiting the use of technology, this option could help prevent inappropriate, harmful, and excessively expensive technologies from being adopted and used. Providers and patients could still use unapproved technologies, but at the price of foregoing Medicare payment. Payment as a force driving the adoption and use of new technologies would be moderated.

This option depends heavily on the existence of evaluative information. Since clinical studies, syntheses, and judgments are all lengthy undertakings, linking third-party payment to more systematic evaluations of technologies could occur only as a gradual, incremental process. Establishing relative efficacy and cost effectiveness as rigid coverage criteria would be impractical (Willems, 1979c). Not all technologies could be subjected to lengthy and costly clinical trials, for example.

Within the Medicare program, the system for triggering the evaluation of a technology is too haphazard to permit uniform application of criteria. Carriers now raise most coverage issues at their own discretion. Many prominent and controversial technologies, such as coronary artery bypass surgery, have not received a review.

Nor could formal evaluative results provide definitive answers about appropriate use to third parties or clinicians (Willems, 1979a). In addition to efficacy, safety, and cost effectiveness, decisions about appropriate use require incorporating social and ethical considerations. And at the level of clinical decisionmaking, circumstances are rarely identical to those in formal analyses. Room must be left for the exercise of clinical judgment.

Third parties could use evaluative results in ways consistent with clinical discretion. The results of clinical trials and cost-effectiveness analyses, for example, could guide extensions of benefits. Studies of primary preventive technologies, such as influenza and pneumococcal vaccines, suggest that some may be cost effective for certain high-risk groups (Kavet, 1972; Willems et al., 1980). Other preventive technologies, such as frequent routine screening for abnormalities, may be less appropriate (Neuhauser and Lewicki, 1976; Schweitzer and Luce, 1978). Evaluations could guide the frequency of use and types of patients that would be covered. Standardized methodology would be needed to permit comparisons of different technologies. Review bodies, such as PSROs, could incorporate formal evaluations into guidelines for physicians, who in turn could be given the opportunity to justify any deviation.

Another option within the context of present financing arrangements is that third parties could base their rates of payment on costs incurred when services are performed efficiently, and on fees designed to encourage the appropriate use of technologies. Medicare and other third parties base their rates of payment on the costs or charges of providers, with little regard for the efficient use of resources to perform a service or for the least costly setting or practitioner. As an alternative, third parties paying an institution's costs could limit payment to the amount of the most efficient method of performing or locating a service. The least expensive method of achieving the desired result could serve as the maximum paid. Such a policy would be consistent with current practices of cost-based payment, such as setting depreciation schedules for equipment. Similarly, fees paid to physicians could reflect desired income levels (Hadley et al., 1979) as well as the desired mix of alternative technologies.

This option would require considerable expertise to set, monitor, and review rates. For both hospitals' and physicians' rates, third parties would require experts with detailed knowledge of such factors as budgets, methods of performing services, and types of equipment. While such attention to rates of payment has the advantage of working within present financing arrangements, it has the disadvantage of perpetuating additional payment for additional services. With rates of payment set, use of technologies and total expenditures may continue to rise.

A more global approach, such as prospective reimbursement, would eliminate the present situation whereby physicians and hospitals are rewarded with higher revenue for performing additional services, regardless of the marginal costs and benefits. Different forms of prospective reimbursement have in common that rates are set in advance of the time period when they apply. The option presented above would set rates of payment. This option would directly or indirectly limit a provider's total revenue—directly through budget review or indirectly through capitation payment.

Limiting total revenue would both enable and force providers to make choices among alternative services and among alternative methods of performing those services. Within the predetermined revenue, a provider could choose which services to perform and how to perform them. Physicians and hospital administrators, rather than third parties, would make the decisions about particular services. The factors that physicians and hospitals weigh when making decisions would undoubtedly undergo great change. Additional services would no longer automatically increase their revenues and might even decrease their incomes by increasing their costs.

This global approach would have the advantage of creating an environment with different incentives without necessitating substantial changes in the way providers are organized. Providers could continue to practice under current arrangements. The altered financial incentives might enhance the competitive position of Health Maintenance Organizations (HMOs), which are already paid by capitation. While organizational change would be possible, it would not be required.

Like the previous option, this one would require technical expertise, in this case to set capitation payments and to review budgets. Moreover, the presence of different incentives would affect the kind of medical care delivered and expenditures only over a long period of time. Continuation of certain regulatory activities would be compatible, if not desirable, under this option. Certificate-of-need and utilization review could help to protect against any tendency by providers to consider costs exclusive of benefits as they operate within fixed revenues. Different forms of this option could be assessed on an experimental basis for the effects on the use of specific technologies, effects on access to technologies, and effects on expenditures for medical care.

Final Thoughts

What did we hope to accomplish in this book?

We wanted above all to bring out the complexity and uncertainty of the subject. We hope to create not a case for doom but rather a case for caution and for the need to know more. Medical technologies must be used appropriately if people are to benefit and are not to be unnecessarily hurt. For that to happen, medicine and its technology must be examined with the best tools that are available or that can be devised. Knowledge about the indications for use of technologies must be increased, and those indications should take into account the health benefits to be gained, the risks to be encountered, and, where appropriate, the costs to be incurred. Further, that use should be examined in the context of social values and impacts.

We hope that we have suggested directions for improvement in the ways that impacts of medical technologies are evaluated and managed. We did not suggest final solutions because we do not feel that these issues are amenable to immediate and final resolution. Society should strive continually to know more about its medical system and technologies. It should systematically seek to understand the incentives leading to appropriate and inappropriate use of technologies.

And finally, we hoped to underscore the complex relationship of medical technology to society. Medicine is part science and technology, part caring and art. Both parts are necessary and both operate within society's cultural, political, economic, and ethical systems. Solutions, therefore, will not come from physicians alone, nor economists, politicians, bureaucrats, ethicists, or anyone, alone. Problems are now being successfully identified through a complex cooperation of disciplines and groups; solutions will only come, gradually, through such effort continued over time.

Appendixes

Appendix A: Office of Technology Assessment— Health Program Reports

This appendix contains brief descriptions of assessments conducted by the Health Program of OTA from its establishment in 1975 to the present. The first report listed was issued in 1974, but it was conducted by OTA health staff.

Drug Bioequivalence

Issued in July of 1974, this was the first report published by OTA. It examined the relationship between the chemical and therapeutic equivalence of drug products.

Development of Medical Technology: Opportunities for Assessment

This report examined the need to assess the social impacts of new medical technologies while they are being developed, the kinds of questions that might be asked in such assessments, by whom, and at what point in the development process assessments could most effectively be conducted. The report presented the case histories of nine technologies to illustrate medical technologies, how they are developed, and why assessing their social impacts might be helpful. It was published in August 1976.

Cancer Testing Technology and Saccharin

In the wake of the decision by the Food and Drug Administration (FDA) to ban the use of saccharin as an artificial sweetener, because of laboratory evidence indicating that it caused cancer in animals, OTA was asked by the Subcommittee on Health and Scientific Research of the Senate Committee on Human Resources to: (1) assess the capacity of current testing methodology to predict the carcinogenic potential of chemicals consumed by humans; (2) evaluate the potential risk of cancer from saccharin for humans; (3) evaluate the benefits of saccharin use, particularly for diabetics and those with special medical problems; and (4) assess the potential availability of alternate artificial sweeteners.

The study, conducted by the OTA staff with technical assistance from an 11 member panel of scientists and medical specialists, commissioned 12 short-term tests of the mutagenicity of saccharin. It marked the first time that scientific experiments were carried out as part of an OTA assessment. The report was published in October 1977.

Policy Implications of Medical Information Systems

This report examined the policy implications of using computer-based information systems for clinical care as well as for business or administrative functions. In addition, the report presented analyses of the benefits and limitations of medical information systems, the factors influencing their adoption, and alternative Federal policies regarding their use. The study was issued in November 1977.

Policy Implications of Computed Tomography (CT) Scanners

The revolutionary nature of CT scanner technology, the speed of its acceptance, and its expense have produced many problems for the medical system. Because many of these problems are common to other new medical technologies, the case study of the CT scanner highlighted several important issues for health policy.

This study examined Federal policy regarding safety and efficacy; the effect of health planning and regulatory policies on diffusion; the relationship between efficacy and patterns of use; and the impact of reimbursement policies on expenditures. It was published in August 1978. An update of this report was issued in 1980.

Assessing the Efficacy and Safety of Medical Technologies

This study further developed issues raised by OTA's report on CT scanners. The study investigated the need for assessing the efficacy and safety of current and future medical technologies. It also discussed the methods and procedures used in evaluating medical technologies. Finally, it described the types of assessment programs currently supported by the Federal Government, and suggested alternatives for improving existing assessment programs and policies. (See Chapter 6 of this book.) The report was released in September of 1978.

Selected Topics in Federal Health Statistics

The Federal Government lacks a coherent policy on the collection, analysis, and use of statistical information regarding people's health and their use of medical care resources. There is currently no national health information system. Instead, there is a patchwork of numerous data collection projects, each of which addresses a different need or purpose. Moreover, there is no systematic appraisal of the adequacy, need for, or use of health data that are currently collected.

This assessment was divided into two parts. One study examined all statutory authorities that require agencies within the (then) Department of Health, Education, and Welfare to collect health data. The other is focused on the lack of coordination among various Federal agencies that collect health data, and it outlined alternatives for integrating health data collection and use. Both parts were issued as one volume in June 1979.

Computer Technology in Medical Education and Assessment

This report reviewed the state-of-the-art of the use of computer technology in medical education and assessment. It described the technologies and strategies for computer-based education and assessment, the current state of medical education and assessment activities, and computer applications in medicine. It also provided examples of systems for the development and dissemination of computer-based educational materials. A summary and analysis of such computer uses were also presented. Although the focus of the report is on physician education and assessment, the implications of the activities described are applicable to other health professions. It was published in September 1979.

A Review of Selected Federal Vaccine and Immunization Policies (Based on Case Studies of Pneumococcal Vaccine)

Using the development of pneumococcal vaccine as a case study, this report identified selected issues in three general areas: vaccine research and development in both the public and private sectors, the cost effectiveness of preventing diseases through the use of vaccines, and factors that affect the use of preventive health technologies in general and vaccines in particular.

This report also analyzed the cost effectiveness of using pneumococcal vaccine as a preventive health measure in selected segments of the population. This vaccine is intended mainly for people who have a high risk of contracting pneumococcal pneumonia. Theoretically, it is more desirable to prevent this form of pneumonia through vaccination than to treat it. Prevention could not only reduce hospital and other treatment costs, but it also could lower the number of deaths caused by pneumonia, the leading killer among infectious diseases in the United States. OTA examined the validity and social implications of this idea.

Finally, this report identified various factors that affect the use of vaccines, such as consumer awareness of benefits and risks, availability and cost, incentives to administer vaccines, liability for harm resulting from vaccination, and government efforts to promote vaccine use. All of these factors need to be considered by public health planners when designing programs, either to help prevent or to help treat disease.

This study was issued in September of 1979.

Cost Effectiveness of Medical Technologies

Cost-effectiveness analysis is often suggested as a way to help allocate health resources more rationally. Such analysis compares the costs of alternate ways of attaining specified goals or effects. There is growing pressure to make cost effectiveness a prime consideration in deciding whether to adopt particular medical technologies, yet we know little about the implications of using this technique widely.

This assessment examined the social costs and benefits of potentially widespread use of cost-effectiveness analysis and cost-benefit analysis in health care decisionmaking. It evaluated: (1) the methodological feasibility of using such analyses; (2) the need for their use; (3) the potential ethical, economic, political, and legal implications of expanded use of these analytical techniques; and (4) the feasibility of properly incorporating results of such analyses into decisionmaking systems. Besides a report addressing the above issues and setting out policy options, the assessment produced a methodology and literature review; a report of an international comparison of use of cost-effectiveness analysis and other mechanisms for managing medical technology; and about 20 case studies of specific medical technologies. This assessment was issued in August 1980.

Technologies for Forecasting Physician Supply and Demand

Several models have been developed and used to predict both the supply of and requirements for physicians. However, these forecasting methods can yield very different estimates, and considerable debate surrounds the interpretation of these results, leaving Congress in doubt about their implications.

The assessment consists of three tasks:

1. Specification of forecasting models. Explicit assumptions used in the models, as well as the results, will be compared in a quick reference format.
2. Technical review of models. The results of each model will be compared to ascertain the relative importance and weighting of model components and underlying assumptions.
3. Implications of predictive models. The implications for policy of relying on different models will be considered. The effects of changing the underlying assumptions on the estimates for the aggregate number, the number of primary care physicians, and for the geographic distribution of physicians will be analyzed.

This study was issued in April 1980.

Technologies for Determining Cancer Risks from the Environment

Prevention of cancer has moved during the past 20 years from a seldom-voiced idea to a prominent aspect of public health thinking. Reducing exposure to agents that cause cancer requires the identification of causative agents, assessment of their potency, and location of sites of exposure. In addition, regulations to reduce exposure must be politically and socially acceptable.

The assessment includes the following parts:

1. Assessment of the estimated risk of cancer from different exposures. Different data sources and different methods for making projections have produced divergent estimates for the risk from each component of human environment—the air and water, the workplace, radiation, personal habits, and diet. The data sources, the methods, and the use of the estimates in public policy discussions and decisionmaking will be examined and compared.
2. Assessment of cancer testing technologies. Technologies used by the Federal Government and the private sector for the identification of carcinogenic chemicals will be analyzed.
3. Assessment of extrapolation techniques. Carcinogenic chemicals are tested in animals and lower life forms. The assessment will analyze existing and potential methods that may be used to translate test results into estimates of potential human hazard.
4. What is "unreasonable risk?" If science were perfect, and society knew that a chemical caused a number of cancers, society might still have a problem. If the chemical is essential and at the same time a risk, what should society do? Unreasonable risk can be defined from a number of perspectives, including public health, legal, economic, and ethical. Comparing, contrasting, and merging these views will provide a foundation for policy decisions about risk.

The assessment was initiated in March, 1979 and is expected to be released early in 1981.

Appendix B: Glossary of Acronyms; Organization Chart (Department of Health and Human Services)

Acronyms can save time and space; they are a useful shorthand—for those who use them almost daily. For those who don't, however, they can be frustrating and confusing. This glossary should ease the frustration a bit, especially in regard to the organization chart in this appendix.

AoA:	Administration on Aging (OHDS)
ADAMHA:	Alcohol, Drug Abuse, and Mental Health Administration (PHS)
BoB:	Bureau of Biologics (FDA)
BCHS:	Bureau of Community Health Services (HSA)
BD:	Bureau of Drugs (FDA)
BHF:	Bureau of Health Facilities Financing, Compliance, and Conversion (HRA)
BHP:	Bureau of Health Planning (HRA)
BHPr:	Bureau of Health Professions (HRA)
BMD:	Bureau of Medical Devices (FDA)
BMS:	Bureau of Medical Services (HSA)
BRH:	Bureau of Radiological Health (FDA)
CBA:	Cost-Benefit Analysis
CDC:	Centers for Disease Control (PHS)
CEA:	Cost-Effectiveness Analysis
CEH:	Center for Environmental Health (CDC)
CHEP:	Center for Health Education and Promotion (CDC)
CID:	Center for Infectious Diseases (CDC)
CON:	Certificate of Need

CPS:	Center for Prevention Services (CDC)
ESRD:	End-Stage Renal Disease, or ESRD Program (HCFA)
FDA:	Food and Drug Aministration (PHS)
HCFA:	Health Care Financing Administration (HHS)
HEW:	U.S. Department of Health, Education, and Welfare (now HHS)
HHS:	U.S. Department of Health and Human Services
HMO:	Health Maintenance Organization
HRA:	Health Resources Administration (PHS)
HSA:	Health Services Administration (PHS) or Health Systems Agency (for health planning)
HSQB:	Health Standards and Quality Bureau (HCFA)
IHS:	Indian Health Service (HSA)
NCHCT:	National Center for Health Care Technology (OASH)
NCHS:	National Center for Health Statistics (OASH)
NCHSR:	National Center for Health Services Research (OASH)
NCI:	National Cancer Institute (NIH)
NHLBI:	National Heart, Lung, and Blood Institute (NIH)
NIAAA:	National Institute on Alcohol Abuse and Alcoholism (ADAMHA)
NIAID:	National Institute of Allergy and Infectious Diseases (NIH)
NICHD:	National Institute of Child Health and Human Development (NIH)
NIDA:	National Institute on Drug Abuse (ADAMHA)
NIH:	National Institutes of Health (PHS)
NIMH:	National Institute of Mental Health (ADAMHA)
NIOSH:	National Institute for Occupational Safety and Health (CDCP)
OASH:	Office of the Assistant Secretary for Health (HHS)
ODPHP:	Office of Disease Prevention and Health Promotion (OASH)
OHDS:	Office of Human Development Services
OHMO:	Office of Health Maintenance Organizations (OASH)
OHRST:	Office of Health Research, Statistics, and Technology (OASH)
OMAR:	Office of Medical Applications of Research (NIH)
OPE:	Office of Planning and Evaluation (OASH)
OTA:	Office of Technology Assessment (U.S. Congress)
PHS:	U.S. Public Health Service (HHS)
PSRO:	Professional Standards Review Organization, or Office of PSRO (HCFA)
TA:	Technology Assessment

Appendix Figure B-1.
Department of Health and Human Services—Organizational Components Involved in Medical Technology.

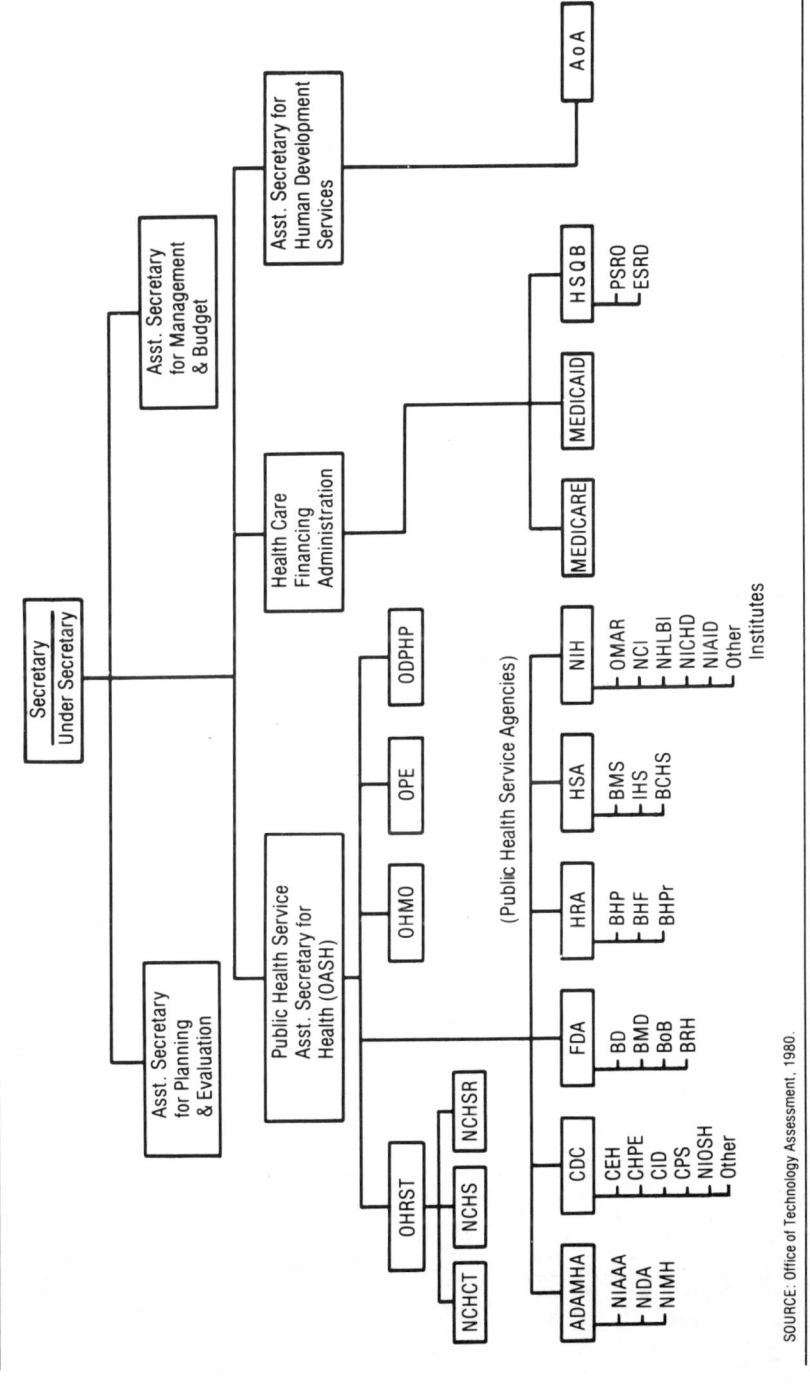

SOURCE: Office of Technology Assessment, 1980.

References/Additional Readings

Abel-Smith, B. Major Patterns of Financing and Organization of Medical Care in Countries Other than the United States. *Bull. New York Acad. Med.* 40: 540, 1964.

Abrams, H. and McNeil, B. Medical Implications of Computed Tomography (CAT Scanning). Parts I and II. *New Eng. J. Med.* 298:255, 310, 1978.

Acton, J. Measuring the Monetary Value of Lifesaving Programs. In *Emergency Medical Services: Research Methodology*. DHEW Publication No. (PHS) 78-3195. Rockville, Maryland: National Center for Health Services Research, 1978.

Alexander, C. The Effects of Change in Methods of Paying the Physician: The Baltimore Experience. *Amer. J. Pub. Health* 57: 1278, 1967.

Altman, S. and Blendon, R. (Eds.). *Medical Technology: The Culprit Behind Health Care Costs?* DHEW Publication No. (PHS) 79-3216. Hyattsville, Maryland: National Center for Health Services Research and Bureau of Health Planning, 1979.

Altman, S. and Wallack, S. Technology on Trial—Is It the Culprit Behind Rising Health Costs? The Case For and Against. In Altman, S. and Blendon, R. (Eds.), *Medical Technology: The Culprit Behind Health Care Costs?* DHEW Publication No. (PHS) 79-3216. Hyattsville, Maryland: National Center for Health Services Research and Bureau of Health Planning, 1979.

American Biology Council. Contributions of the Biological Sciences to Human Welfare. *Federation Proceedings Volume 31* (Part 2), November–December, 1972.

American Hospital Association. *Hospitals Statistics. 1978 Edition*. Chicago, Illinois, 1978a.

American Medical Association. *Health Care Issues: Physician and Public Attitudes*. Compiled from Studies Conducted by the Gallup Organization, Inc. Chicago, Illinois, 1978.

*NOTE: One purpose of this bibliography is to serve as a resource for those interested in the field of medical technology and health policy. Accordingly, we have included not only those sources referenced in the text but also some other publications that are important to the field.

Annerstedt, J. *On the Present Global Distribution of R&D Resources*. Vienna, Austria: Vienna Institute for Development, 1979.

Applied Management Sciences. *Analysis of Prospective Reimbursement Systems: Western Pennsylvania*. Prepared for the Office of Research and Statistics, Department of Health, Education, and Welfare, 1975. Quoted in Wagner, J., *Impact of Hospital Reimbursement Policy*. Project Proposal to the Health Care Financing Administration, Grant 18–P–97113/3–01, 1978.

Arnstein, S. Technology Assessment: Opportunities and Obstacles. *IEEE Transactions on Systems, Man, and Cybernetics* SMC–7:571, 1977.

Arnstein, S. and Christakis, A. *Prespectives on Technology Assessment*. Jerusalem: Science and Technology Publishers, 1975.

Arrow, K. Uncertainty and the Welfare Economics of Medical Care. *American Economic Review* 53:941, 1963.

Avery, A. et al. *Quality of Medical Care Assessment Using Outcome Measures: Eight Disease-Specific Applications*. Santa Monica, California: Rand, 1976.

Bailar, J. Mammography: A Time for Caution. *JAMA*, 237:997, 1977.

Banta, D. The Diffusion of the Computed Tomography (CT) Scanner in the United States. *Int. J. Health Services* 10:251, 1980a.

Banta, D. Computed Tomography: Cost Containment Misdirected. *Amer. J. Pub. Health* 70:215, 1980b.

Banta, D. Abraham Flexner—A Reappraisal. *Soc. Sci. Med.* 5:655, 1971.

Banta, D. and Behney, C. Medical Technology: Policies and Problems. *Health Care Management Review* (In Press).

Banta, D. and Bosch, S. Organized Labor and the Prepaid Group Practice Movement. *Arch. Environmental Health* 29:43, 1974.

Banta, D. and McNeil, B. Evaluation of the CAT Scanner and Other Diagnostic Technologies. *Health Care Management Review* 3:7, 1978.

Banta, D. and Sanes, J. Assessing the Social Impacts of Medical Technologies. *J. Community Health* 3:245, 1978a.

Banta, D. and Sanes, J. How the Cat Got Out of the Bag. In Egdahl, R. and Gertman, P. (Eds.), *Technology and the Quality of Health Care*. Germantown, Maryland: Aspen Systems Corporation, 1978b.

Banta, D. and Thacker, S. Assessing the Costs and Benefits of Electronic Fetal Monitoring. *Obstet. Gyn. Survey* 34(Suppl.):627, 1979a.

Banta, D. and Thacker, S. Policies Toward Medical Technology: The Case of Electronic Fetal Monitoring. *Amer. J. Pub. Health* 69:931, 1979b.

Banta, D. et al., Weighing the Benefits and Costs of Medical Technologies. *Proc. IEEE* 67:1190, 1979.

Banta, D. et al. Implications of the 1976 Medical Devices Legislation. *Man and Medicine* 3:131, 1978.

Barach, A. and Segal, M. The Indiscriminate Use of IPPB. *JAMA* 231:1141, 1975.

Barber, B. The Ethics of Experimentation with Human Subjects. *Scientific American* 234:25, 1976.

Barker-Benfield, G. *The Horrors of the Half-Known Life*. New York: Harper and Row, 1976.

Baroon, S. and Wolfe, H. *Measuring the Effectiveness of Medical Decisions*. Springfield, Illinois: Charles C Thomas, 1972.

Barsamian, E. The Rise and Fall of Internal Mammary Artery Ligation in the Treatment of Angina and the Lessons Learned. In Bunker, J. et al. (Eds.), *Costs, Risks and Benefits of Surgery*. New York: Oxford University Press, 1977.

Batelle. *Interactions of Science and Technology in the Innovative Process: Some Case Studies*. Prepared for the National Science Foundation. Columbus, Ohio: Batelle Columbus Laboratories, 1973.

Batelle Columbus Laboratories. Analysis of Selected Biomedical Research Programs. In *Report of the President's Biomedical Research Panel*. DHEW Publication No. (OS) 76–502, Appendix B. Washington, D.C.: Department of Health, Education, and Welfare, 1976.

Beecher, H. Ethics and Clinical Research. *New Eng. J. Med. 274*:1354, 1966.

Behney, C. *Studies of the Implications of New Medical Technologies*. Rockville, Maryland: Health Resources Administration, Department of Health, Education, and Welfare, 1976.

Behney, C. *In Search of a Demography of Ethics*. (Manuscript.) Washington, D.C.: The George Washington University, 1974.

BEIR Report. *The Effects on Populations of Exposure to Low Levels of Ionizing Radiation*. Report of the Advisory Committee on the Biological Effects of Ionizing Radiations. Washington, D.C.: National Academy of Sciences, 1972.

Bell, R. and Loop, J. The Utility and Futility of Radiographic Skull Examination for Trauma. *New Eng. J. Med. 284*:236, 1971.

Bennett, I. Technology as a Shaping Force. *Daedalus 106*:125, 1977.

Bice, T. et al. *Executive Summary of the Conference on Capital Financing for Health Facilities*. Sponsored by Health Resources Administration and University of Pittsburgh. Pittsburgh, Pennsylvania, Nov. 19–21, 1976.

Blanpain, J. and Deleise, L. *Community Health Investment, Health Services Research in Belgium, France, Federal German Republic and the Netherlands*. London: Oxford University Press, 1976.

Blanpain, J. et al. *International Approaches to Health Resources Development for National Health Programs, Executive Summary of the Study*. Hyattsville, Maryland: Health Resources Administration, Department of Health, Education, and Welfare, 1976.

Boston Women's Health Book Collective. *Our Bodies Ourselves*. New York: Simon & Schuster, 1976.

Braunwald, E. Coronary-Artery Surgery at the Crossroads. *New Eng. J. Med. 297*:661, 1977.

Breslow, L. Basic Issues in Biomedical Research. Testimony Before the Subcommittee on Health, Committee on Labor and Public Welfare, United States Senate, Washington, D.C., June 17, 1976.

Broida, J. Medical Technology in Japan. Draft Paper for the Office of Technology Assessment, Congress of the United States, Washington, D.C., 1979.

Brook, R. Controlling the Use and Cost of Medical Services: The New Mexico

Experimental Medical Care Review Organization—A Four Year Case Study. *Medical Care 16*(Suppl.), September, 1978.
Brook, R. Quality of Care Assessment: Policy Relevant Issues. *Policy Sciences* 5:317, 1974.
Brook, R. *Quality of Care Assessment: A Comparison of Five Methods of Peer Review.* Washington, D.C.: National Center for Health Services Research, Department of Health, Education, and Welfare, 1973.
Brook, R. and Appel, F. Quality of Care Assessment: Choosing a Method for Peer Review. *New Eng. J. Med. 288*:1323, 1973.
Brook, R. and Williams, K. Evaluation of the New Mexico Peer Review System 1971 to 1973. *Medical Care 14*(Suppl.), December, 1976.
Brook, R. et al. Assessing the Quality of Medical Care Using Outcome Measures: An Overview of the Method. *Medical Care 15*(Suppl.), September, 1977.
Brook, R. et al. *Quality of Medical Care Assessment Using Health Outcome Measures: An Overview of the Method.* Prepared for the National Center for Health Services Research. Santa Monica, California: Rand, 1976.
Brown, J. and Dickson, J. Instrumentation and the Delivery of Health Services. *Science 166*:334, 1969.
Brown, S. *Policy Issues in the Health Sciences.* Washington, D.C.: Institute of Medicine, National Academy of Sciences, 1977.
Brownfield, R. and Ives, E. Creating a Data Base for the Laboratory Universe. *Lab. Management 14*:22, 1976.
Bunker, J. Surgical Manpower. A Comparison of Operations and Surgeons in the United States and in England and Wales. *New Eng. J. Med. 282*:135, 1970.
Bunker, J. et al. (Eds.). *Costs, Risks and Benefits of Surgery.* New York: Oxford University Press, 1977.
Burkhardt, R. and Kienle, G. Controlled Clinical Trials and Medical Ethics. *Lancet* 2:1356, 1978.
Byar, D. et al. Randomized Clinical Trials. *New Eng. J. Med. 295*:74, 1976.
Carter, G. et al. Policy Analysis for Federal Biomedical Research. In *Report of the President's Biomedical Research Panel.* DHEW Publication No. (OS) 76-502, Appendix B. Washington, D.C.: Department of Health, Education, and Welfare, 1976.
Cauffman, J. et al. The Impact of Health Insurance Coverage on Health Care of School Children. *Pub. Health Reports 82*:323, 1967.
Chalmers, I. and Lawson, J. Evaluation of Different Approaches to Obstetric Care: Part 1. *Br. J. Obstet. Gyn. 83*:921, 1976.
Chalmers, I. and Richards, M. Intervention and Causal Inference in Obstetric Practice. In Chard, T. and Richards, M. (Eds.), *Benefits and Hazards of the New Obstetrics.* London: Heinemann Medical Books, 1977.
Chalmers, T. Settling the UGDP Controversy. *JAMA 231*:624, 1975.
Chalmers, T. et al. Controlled Studies in Clinical Cancer Research. *New Eng. J. Med. 287*:75, 1972.
Childs, A. and Hunter, D. Non-Medical Factors Influencing Use of Diagnostic X-ray by Physicians. *Med. Care 10*:323, 1972.

Cleeman, J. Coverage Recommendations by the Public Health Service. Washington, D.C.: National Center for Health Care Technology, Department of Health, Education, and Welfare, 1979.

Coates, J. Technology Assessment: The Benefits . . . The Costs . . . The Consequences. *Futurist* 5:225, 1971.

Coates, V. *Technology and Public Policy. Summary Report*. Washington, D.C.: The George Washington University, Program of Policy Studies in Science & Technology, 1972.

Cochrane, A. *Effectiveness and Efficiency*. Abingdon, England: Burgess & Son, 1972.

Coleman, J. et al. *Medical Innovation: A Diffusion Study*. Indianapolis, Indiana: Bobbs-Merrill, 1966.

Colle, A. and Grossman, M. Determinants of Pediatric Care Utilization. *J. Human Resources* 13 (Suppl.):115, 1978.

Colombo, F. et al. *Epidemiological Evaluation of Drugs*. Amsterdam: Elsevier/North Holland Biomedical Press, 1977.

Committee on the Life Sciences and Social Policy. *Assessing Biomedical Technologies: An Inquiry into the Nature of the Process*. Washington, D.C.: National Academy of Sciences, 1975.

Committee on Technology and Health Care. *Medical Technology and the Health Care System*. Washington, D.C.: National Academy of Sciences, 1979.

Comroe, J. and Dripps, R. Scientific Basis for the Support of Biomedical Science. *Science* 192:105, 1976.

Comroe, J. and Dripps, R. Ben Franklin and Open Heart Surgery. *Circ. Res.* 35:661, 1974.

Congressional Budget Office. *The Effect of PSROs on Health Care Costs: Current Findings and Future Evaluations*. Washington, D.C.: GPO, 1979.

Congressional Budget Office. *Expenditures for Health Care: Federal Programs and Their Effects*. Washington, D.C.: GPO, 1977.

Cooper, B. and Gaus, C. Controlling Health Technology. In Altman, S. and Blendon, R. (Eds.), *Medical Technology: The Culprit Behind Health Care Costs?* DHEW Publication No. (PHS) 79–3216. Hyattsville, Maryland: National Center for Health Services Research and Bureau of Health Planning, 1979.

Cooper, J. *The Philosophy of Evidence*. Washington, D.C.: Interdisciplinary Communication Associations, Inc., 1972.

Cooper, J. *Decision-Making on the Efficacy and Safety of Drugs: Philosophy and Technology of Drug Assessment (Vol. I)*. Washington, D.C.: Interdisciplinary Communication Associates, Inc., 1971.

Corbin, M. and Krute, A. Some Aspects of Medicare Experience with Group-Practice Prepayment Plans. *Soc. Sec. Bull.* 38:3, 1975.

Cousins, N. Anatomy of an Illness (as Perceived by the Patient). *New Eng. J. Med.* 295:1458, 1976.

Cromwell, J. et al. *Incentives and Decisions Underlying Hospitals' Adoption and Utilization of Major Capital Equipment*. Report to National Center for Health Services Research and Development, U.S. Department of Health, Education, and Welfare. Cambridge, Massachusetts: ABT Associates, 1975.

Davis, K. The Role of Technology, Demand and Labor Markets in the Determination of Hospital Costs. In Perlman, M. (Ed.), *The Economics of Health and Medical Care*. New York: John Wiley & Sons, 1974.

Deane, R. T. et al. *A Feasibility Study of the Influence of Capital Expenditures on Hospital Operating Costs*. DHEW Contract No. (SSA) 230-76-0260, Task Order No. 33. Silver Spring, Maryland: Applied Management Sciences, 1978.

Delbanco, R. et al. Paying the Physician's Fee. *New Eng. J. Med.* 301:1314, 1979.

Department of Health, Education, and Welfare. Health Planning National Guidelines. *Federal Register* 43:13040, March 28, 1978a.

Department of Health, Education, and Welfare. *DHEW Health Research Principles. Volume I, Documents Relating to the Development of Draft Health Research Principles for the Department of Health, Education, and Welfare, April–December 1978*. DHEW Publication No. (NIH) 79–1890. Washington, D.C., 1978b.

Department of Health, Education, and Welfare. *Report of the Secretary's Commission on Medical Malpractice*. DHEW Publication No. (OS) 73–88. Washington, D.C., 1973.

Diehr, P. et al. Utilization: Ambulatory and Hospital. In *The Seattle Prepaid Health Care Project: Comparison of Health Services Delivery*. Seattle: University of Washington, 1976. Quoted in Luft, H., Why Do HMO's Seem to Provide More Health Maintenance Services? *MMFQ/Health and Society* 56:140, 1978.

Donabedian, A. *Needed Research in the Assessment and Monitoring of the Quality of Medical Care*. DHEW Publication No. (PHS) 78–3219. Washington, D.C.: National Center for Health Services Research, 1978a.

Donabedian, A. The Quality of Medical Care: Methods for Assessing and Monitoring the Quality of Care for Research and for Quality Assurance Programs. In *Health United States*. DHEW Publication No. (PHS) 78–1232. Washington, D.C.: Department of Health, Education, and Welfare, 1978b.

Donabedian, A. *A Guide to Medical Care Administration. II. Medical Care Appraisal—Quality and Utilization*. New York: American Public Health Association, 1969.

Donabedian, A. Evaluating the Quality of Medical Care. *Milbank Memorial Fund Quarterly* 44:169, 1966.

Donabedian, A. *A Review of Some Experiences with Prepaid Group Practice*. Research Series No. 12. Ann Arbor: School of Public Health, University of Michigan, 1965.

Doty, P. Memo to the Interstate and Foreign Commerce Committee. Washington, D.C.: Office of Technology Assessment, March, 1980.

Dowling, H. *Medicines for Man*. New York: Alfred A Knopf, 1970.

Dowling, W. et al. Prospective Reimbursement in Downstate New York and Its Impact in Hospitals—A Summary. University of Washington, 1976. Quoted in Wagner, J., *Impact of Hospital Reimbursement Policy*. Project Proposal to the Health Care Financing Administration, Grant 18–P–97113/3–01, 1978.

Downs, G. and Mohr, L. Conceptual Issues in the Study of Innovation. *Administrative Science Quarterly* 21:700, 1976.

Dumbaugh, K. Policy for Medical Technology in Germany. Draft Paper for the Office of Technology Assessment, Congress of the United States, Washington, D.C., 1979.

Ebert, R. Medical Education in the United States. *Daedalus* 106:171, 1977.

Ebert, R. Use of Anticoagulants in Acute Myocardial Infarction. *Circulation* 45:903, 1972.

Eden, H. and Eden, M. *The Use of Microprocessor-Based "Intelligent" Machines in Patient Care.* NIH Publication No. 79–1852. Washington, D.C.: Department of Health, Education, and Welfare, 1979.

Ehrenreich, B. and English, D. *For Her Own Good.* Garden City, N.Y.: Anchor Press, 1979.

Elliott, D. and Elliott, R. *The Control of Technology.* London: Wykeham Publications Ltd., 1976.

Ellul, J. *The Technological Society.* Translated from the 1954 French edition by John Wilkinson. New York: Random House, 1964.

Ellwood, P. et al. *Assuring the Quality of Health Care.* Minneapolis, Minnesota: Interstudy, 1973.

Enthoven, A. and Noll, R. Regulatory and Nonregulatory Strategies for Controlling Health Care Costs. In Altman, S. and Blendon, R. (Eds.), *Medical Technology: The Culprit Behind Health Care Costs?* DHEW Publication No. (PHS) 79–3216. Hyattsville, Maryland: National Center for Health Services Research and Bureau of Health Planning, 1979.

Evans, R. Does Canada Have too Many Doctors?—Why Nobody Loves an Immigrant Physician. *Canadian Public Policy* 2:147, 1976.

Evans, R. Supplier-Induced Demand: Some Empirical Evidence and Implications. In Perlman, M. (Ed.), *The Economics of Health and Medical Care.* New York: John Wiley and Sons, 1974.

Evans, R. et al. Medical Productivity, Scale Effects and Demand Generation. *Canadian J. Econ.* 6:376, 1973.

Fein, R. But on the Other Hand. *New Eng. J. Med.* 296:751, 1977.

Fein, R. *The Doctor Shortage: An Economic Diagnosis.* Washington, D.C.: The Brookings Institution, 1967.

Fein, R. *Economics of Mental Illness.* Report to the Staff Director, Joint Commission on Mental Illness and Health, Monograph Series No. 2. New York: Basic Books, Inc., 1958.

Fein, R. and Bishop C. *Employment Impacts of Health Policy Developments.* Special Report No. 11. Washington, D.C.: National Commission for Manpower Policy, 1976.

Feinstein, A. Clinical Biostatistics. XXV. A Survey of the Statistical Procedures in General Medical Journals. *Clin. Pharm. Therapeut.* 15:97, 1974.

Feldstein, M. *The Rising Cost of Hospital Care.* Washington, D.C.: Information Resources Press, 1971.

Feldstein, M. and Taylor, A. *The Rapid Rise of Hospital Costs*. Washington, D.C.: President's Council on Wage and Price Stability, 1977.

Fineberg, H. Gastric Freezing—A Study of Diffusion of a Medical Innovation. In Committee on Technology and Health Care, *Medical Technology and the Health Care System*. Washington, D.C.: National Academy of Sciences, 1979.

Fineberg, H. and Hiatt, H. Evaluation of Medical Practices. *New Eng. J. Med.* 301:1086, 1979.

Fineberg, H. et al. Computerized Cranial Tomography: Effect on Diagnostic and Therapeutic Plans. *JAMA* 238:224, 1977a.

Fineberg, H. et al. CT Scanners: Distribution and Planning in the United States. *New Eng. J. Med.* 297:216, 1977b.

Fletcher, J. *Situation Ethics: The New Morality*. Philadelphia: The Westminster Press, 1975.

Fletcher, R. and Fletcher, S. Clinical Research in General Medical Journals. *New Eng. J. Med.* 301:180, 1979.

Fox, R. Advanced Medical Technology—Social and Ethical Implications. In Fox, R., *Essays in Medical Sociology: Journeys into the Field*. New York: John Wiley & Sons, Inc., 1979a.

Fox, R. Ethical and Existential Developments in Contemporaneous American Medicine: Their Implications for Culture and Society. In Fox, R., *Essays in Medical Sociology: Journeys into the Field*. New York: John Wiley & Sons, Inc., 1979b.

Fox, R. Medical Evolution. In Fox, R., *Essays in Medical Sociology: Journeys into the Field*. New York: John Wiley & Sons, Inc., 1979c.

Fox, R. The Medicalization and Demedicalization of American Society. In Fox, R., *Essays in Medical Sociology: Journeys into the Field*. New York: John Wiley & Sons, Inc. 1979d.

Fox, R. The Medical Profession's Changing Outlook on Hemodialysis (1950–1976). In Fox, R., *Essays in Medical Sociology: Journeys into the Field*. New York: John Wiley & Sons, Inc., 1979e.

Fox, R. Organ Transplantation: Sociocultural Aspects. In Fox, R., *Essays in Medical Sociology: Journeys into the Field*. New York: John Wiley & Sons, Inc., 1979f.

Fox, R. and Swazey, J. Kidney Dialysis and Transplantation. In Fox, R., *Essays in Medical Sociology: Journeys into the Field*. New York: John Wiley & Sons, Inc., 1979.

Fox, R. and Swazey, J. *The Courage to Fail*. Chicago: University of Chicago Press, 1974.

Frazier, H. and Hiatt, H. Evaluation of Medical Practices. *Science* 200: 875, 1978.

Fredrickson, D. Health and the Search for New Knowledge. *Daedalus* 106:159, 1977.

Freeborn, D. et al. Determinants of Medical Care Utilization: Physicians' Use of Laboratory Services. *Amer. J. Pub. Health* 62:846, 1972.

Freymann, J. *The American Health Care System: Its Genesis and Trajectory*. New York: Medcom Press, 1974.

Friedson, E. *Profession of Medicine*. New York: Dodd, Mead & Co., 1970.
Friedson, E. *Patient's Views of Medical Practice*. New York: Russell Sage Foundation, 1961.
Frost, S. et al. *A Consumer's Guide to Evaluating Medical Technology*. New York: Consumer Commission on the Accreditation of Health Services, 1979.
Fruen, M. An Overview of the Medical Education System and Its Financing. In Hadley, J. (Ed.), *Medical Education Financing: Policy Analyses and Options for the 1980s*. New York: Prodist, 1980, pp. 23–25.
Fuchs, V. From Bismarck to Woodcock: The 'Irrational' Pursuit of National Health Insurance. Center for Economic Analysis of Human Behavior and Social Institutions, Working Paper No. 120. New York: National Bureau of Economic Research, 1976.
Fuchs, V. *Who Shall Live?*. New York: Basic Books, 1974.
Fuchs, V. and Kramer, M. *Determinants of Expenditures for Physicians' Services in the United States 1948–68*. DHEW Publication No. (HSM) 73–3013. Rockville, Maryland: National Center for Health Services Research and Development, 1972.
Fuhrer, R. Policy for Medical Technology in France. Draft Paper for the Office of Technology Assessment, Congress of the United States, Washington, D.C., 1979.
Futures Group, Inc. *A Study of Life Extending Technologies*, (Volumes 1–6). Glastonbury, Connecticut, 1977.
Gaensler, E. et al. International Project on Health Care Systems and Medical Technology, Sweden. Draft Paper for the Office of Technology Assessment, Congress of the United States, Washington, D.C., 1979.
Galbraith, J. *The New Industrial State*. New York: The New American Library, Inc., 1977.
Gaus, C. Biomedical Research and Health Care Costs. Testimony Before the President's Biomedical Research Panel, Washington, D.C., September 29, 1975.
Gaus, C. and Cooper, B. Technology and Medicare: Alternatives for Change. In Egdahl, R. and Gertman, P. (Eds.), *Technology and the Quality of Health Care*. Germantown, Maryland: Aspen Systems Corporation, 1978.
Gaus, C. et al. Contrasts in HMO and Fee-for-Service Performance. *Soc. Sec. Bull.* 39:3, 1976.
Gelfand, M. Tax-Exempt Financing for Hospital Investment. In Russell, L., *Technology in Hospitals: Medical Advances and Their Diffusion*. Report to the National Science Foundation. Washington, D.C.: The Brookings Institution, 1978.
Gibson, R. and Fisher, C. National Health Expenditures, Fiscal Year 1977. *Soc. Sec. Bull.* 41:3, 1978.
Ginsburg, P. Resource Allocation in the Hospital Industry: The Role of Capital Financing. *Soc. Sec. Bull.* 35:20, 1972.
GMENAC (Graduate Medical Education National Advisory Commmittee). *Interim Report of the Graduate Medical Education National Advisory Committee to the Secretary*. DHEW Publication No. (HRA) 79–633. Hyattsville, Maryland: Department of Health, Education, and Welfare, 1979, Table 2.

Gordon, G. and Fisher, G. *The Diffusion of Medical Technology*. Cambridge, Mass.: Ballinger Publishing Company, 1975.
Gore, S. et al. Misuse of Statistical Methods: Critical Assessment of Articles in BMJ from January to March 1976. *Br. Med. J. 1*:85, 1977.
Government of Quebec. *Report of the Commission of Inquiry on Health and Social Welfare*, Part 2, Vol. IV, Tome III. 1970, pp. 108–112.
Greenberg, B. Conduct of Cooperative Field and Clinical Trials. *Amer. Statistician 13*:13, 1959.
Greer, A. Advances in the Study of Diffusion and Innovation in Health Care Organizations. *MMFQ/Health and Society, 55*:505, 1977a.
Greer, A. Hospital Adoption of Medical Technology: A Preliminary Investigation into Hospital Decisonmaking. Milwaukee: Urban Research Center, University of Wisconsin, 1977b.
Griliches, Z. Hybrid Corn: An Exploration in the Economics of Technological Change. *Econometrica 25*:501, 1957.
Griner, P. Treatment of Acute Pulmonary Edema: Conventional or Intensive Care? *Ann. of Intern. Med. 77*:501, 1972.
Groot, L. The Dutch Health Care System and Its Relation to Medical Technology. Draft Paper for the Office of Technology Assessment, Congress of the United States, Washington, D.C., 1979.
Grosse, R. Cost-Benefit Analysis of Health Services. *Ann. Amer. Acad. Polit. Soc. Science 399*:89, 1972.
Gunnarson, D. and Neuhauser, D. International Project on Health Care Systems and Medical Technology. Draft Paper for the Office of Technology Assessment, Congress of the United States, Washington, D.C., 1979.
Hadley, J. et al. Can Fee-for-Service Reimbursement Coexist with Demand Creation? *Inquiry 16*:247, 1979.
Handler, P. *Biology and the Future of Man*. New York: Oxford University Press, 1970.
Hanft, R. et al. *Hospital Cost Containment*. New York: Prodist (for the Milbank Memorial Fund), 1978.
Harris, J. The Internal Organization of Hospitals: Some Economic Implications. *Bell J. Econ. 8*:467, 1977.
Hastings, J. et al. Prepaid Group Practice in Sault Ste. Marie, Ontario: Part I: Analysis of Utilization Records. *Medical Care 11*:91, 1973.
Hatcher, P. Hospital Cost Containment Approaches in Ontario. Presented at the Meeting of the American Public Health Association, New York, November 5, 1979.
Health Care Financing Administration (HCFA). PRSO Hospital Review: Relationship of PSRO to Hospitals and Use of Hospital Review Committees; Norms for PSRO Hospital Review. Regulation on the PSRO Program, 42 CFR, Part 466. *Federal Register 44*:32074, June 4, 1979.
Health Insurance Institute. *Health and Health Insurance: The Public's View*. Washington, D.C., 1979.

Health Technology Management at the Department of Health, Education, and Welfare, Final Phase I Report for the Secretary, Washington, D.C., December 22, 1977.

Hetman, F. *Society and the Assessment of Technology.* Paris: The Organization for Economic Cooperation and Development, 1973.

Hiatt, H. "Protecting the Medical Commons: Who Is Responsible?" *New England Journal of Medicine,* 293, 235, 1975.

Hill, B. *Principles of Medical Statistics.* New York: Oxford University Press, 1971.

Hill, B. *Statistical Methods in Clinical and Preventive Medicine.* London: E. & S. Livingston, Ltd., 1962.

Hill, B. The Clinical Trial. *New Eng. J. Med.* 247:113, 1952.

Hill, B. *Medical Statistics.* Edinburgh, Scotland: R & R Clark, Ltd., 1937.

Hollis, G. *State Licensing of Health Facilities.* Washington, D.C.: National Center for Health Statistics, Department of Health, Education, and Welfare, 1968.

House of Representatives. Committee on Interstate and Foreign Commerce. *Investigation of the National Institutes of Health.* Washington, D.C.: GPO, 1976a.

House of Representatives. Subcomittee on Oversight and Investigations, Committee on Interstate and Foreign Commerce. *Cost and Quality of Health Care: Unnecessary Surgery.* Washington, D.C.: GPO, 1976b.

House of Representatives. Committee on Interstate and Foreign Commerce. *Getting Ready for National Health Insurance: Unnecessary Surgery.* Hearings Before the Subcommittee on Health and the Environment. Washington, D.C.: GPO, 1975.

Hutt, P. Balanced Government Regulation of Consumer Products. Rochester, N.Y.: Center for the Study of Drug Development, University of Rochester Medical Center, Publications Series PS–7601, Fall, 1976.

Hypertension Detection and Follow-up Program Cooperative Group. Five-Year Findings of the Hypertension Detection and Follow-up Program. 1. Reduction in Mortality of Persons with High Blood Pressure, Including Mild Hypertension. *JAMA* 242:2562, 1979.

Iglehart, J. The Cost and Regulation of Medical Technology: Future Policy Directions. *MMFQ/Health and Society* 55:25, 1977.

Illich, I. *Medical Nemesis: The Expropriation of Health.* New York: Pantheon Books, Random House, Inc., 1976.

Institute of Medicine, National Academy of Sciences. *DHEW's Research Planning Principles: A Review.* Publication No. (NIH) 79–1955. Washington, D.C.: Department of Health, Education, and Welfare, 1979.

Institute of Medicine. *A Manpower Policy for Primary Care.* Washington, D.C.: National Academy of Sciences, 1978.

Institute of Medicine. *Assessing Quality in Health Care: An Evaluation.* Washington, D.C.: National Academy of Sciences, 1976.

Institute of Medicine. *Advancing the Quality of Health Care.* Washington, D.C.: National Academy of Sciences, 1974.

Jonas, S. *Medical Mystery.* New York: W.W. Norton & Company, 1978.

Jonas, S. Measurement and Control of Health Care Quality. In Jonas, S. (Ed.), *Health Care Delivery in the United States*. New York: Springer Publishing Company, 1977.

Johnson, E. Letter. *New Eng. J. Med.* 299:665, 1978.

Jonsson, E. and Marke, L. CAT Scanner: The Swedish Experience. *Health Care Management Review* 1:37, 1977.

Joseph, H. Empirical Research on the Demand for Medical Care. *Inquiry* 8:61, 1971.

Kaluzny, A. Innovation in Health Services: Theoretical Framework and Review of Research. *Health Services Research* 9:101, 1974.

Kaluzny, A. et al. Health Systems. In Gordon, G. and Fisher, L. (Eds.), *The Diffusion of Medical Technology*. Cambridge, Mass.: Ballinger Publishing Co., 1975.

Kaluzny, A. et al. Innovation of Health Services: A Comparative Study of Hospitals and Health Departments. *MMFQ/Health and Society* 52:51, 1974.

Kamien, M. and Schwartz, N. Market Structure and Innovation: A Survey. *J. Econ. Literature* 13:1, 1975.

Kavet, J. Influenza and Public Policy. Unpublished Doctoral Thesis. Cambridge, Mass., Harvard University, School of Public Health, 1972.

Kelling, R. and Williams, P. The Projected Response of the Capital Market to Health Facilities Expenditures for the Years 1976–1981. Presented at the Conference on Capital Financing for Health Facilities, Pittsburgh, Pennsylvania, November 19–21, 1976.

Kennedy, C. and Thirlwell, A. Survey in Applied Economics: Technical Progress. *Econ. J.* 82:11, 1972.

Kessner, D. and Kalk, C. *Contrasts in Health Status, 2: A Strategy for Evaluating Health Services*. Washington, D.C.: Institute of Medicine, National Academy of Sciences, 1973.

Kessner, D. et al. Assessing Health Quality—The Case for Tracers. *New Eng. J. Med.* 288:189, 1973.

Kimbell, L. and Lorant, J. Physician Productivity and Returns to Scale. *Health Services Research* 12:367, 1977.

Kimerbly, J. Hospital Adoption of Innovations in Medical and Managerial Technology: Individual Organization and Contextual/Environmental Effects. Final Project Report for the National Science Foundation, Yale University, March 1978.

Klarman, H. Application of Cost-Benefit Analysis to the Health Services and the Special Case of Technology. *Intl. J. Health Services* 4:325, 1974.

Klarman, H. Observations on Health Care Technology: Measurement, Analysis, and Policy. In Altman, S. and Blendon, R. (Eds.), *Medical Technology: The Culprit Behind Health Care Costs?* DHEW Publication No. (PHS) 79-3216. Hyattsville, Maryland: National Center for Health Services Research and Bureau of Health Planning, 1979.

Klarman, H. and Guzick, D. Economics of Influenza. In Selby, P. (Ed.), *Influenza—Virus, Vaccines, and Strategy: Proceedings of a Working Group on Pandemic Influenza*. New York: Academic Press, 1976.

Klarman, H. et al. Cost-Effectiveness Analysis Applied to the Treatment of Chronic Renal Disease. *Medical Care* 6:48, 1968.
Klein, R. The Rise and Decline of Policy Analysis: The Strange Case of Health Policy Making in Britain. *Policy Analysis* 2:459, 1976.
Knatterud, G. et al. Effects of Hypoglycemic Agents on Vascular Complications in Patients with Adult-Onset Diabetes. *JAMA* 217:777, 1971.
Knowles, J. The Hospital. *Scientific American* 229:128, 1973.
Kron, J. Did the Girl in the Coma Want 'Death with Dignity'? *New York* 8:60, 1975.
Lairson, D. and Swint, J. A Multivariate Analysis of the Likelihood and Volume of Preventive Visits Demand in a Prepaid Group Practice. *Medical Care* 11:730, 1978.
Lambert, E.C. *Modern Medical Mistakes*. Bloomington, Indiana: Indiana University Press, 1978.
Lampert, R. et al. A Critical Look at Oral Decongestants. *Pediatrics* 55:550, 1975.
Lee, R. and Jones, L. *The Fundamentals of Good Medical Care*. Chicago: The University of Chicago Press, 1933.
Lembcke, P. Medical Auditing by Scientific Methods. *JAMA* 162:646, 1956.
Lewin and Associates, Inc. *Evaluation of the Efficiency and Effectiveness of the Section 1122 Review Process*. Report to Health Resources Administration, U.S. Department of HEW, Contract No. HRA-106-74-183. Washington, D.C.: Lewin and Associates, Inc., September 1975.
Lewis, C. Variations in the Incidence of Surgery. *New Eng. J. Med.* 281:880, 1969.
Lewis, C. and Keairnes, H. Controlling Costs of Medical Care by Expanding Insurance Coverage. *New Eng. J. Med.* 282:1405, 1970.
Levy, R. Implications of the Innovative Process and of Impact Assessment on the Management of Biomedical Research. Presented at the Meeting on Development and Dissemination of Biomedical Innovations: Foundations for Program Development, Mt. Pocono, Pennsylvania, March 17-19, 1980.
LoGerfo, J. Necessity of Care: Definitions and Issues. Presented at the Meeting of the American Public Health Association, New York, November 6, 1979.
Lowrance, W. *Of Acceptable Risk*. Los Altos, California: William Kaufmann, Inc., 1976.
Luft, H. HMO's and Medical Costs: The Rhetoric and the Evidence. *New Eng. J. Med.* 298:1336, 1978.
Luft, H. Benefit-Cost Analysis and Public Policy Implementation: From Normative to Positive Analysis. *Public Policy* 24:437, 1976.
Lusted, L. et al. Evaluating the Efficacy of Radiologic Procedures by Bayesian Methods: A Progress Report. In Snapper, K. (Ed.), *Models in Metrics for Decision Makers*. Washington, D.C.: Information Resources Press, (In Press).
McCann, J. and Ames, B. Detection of Carcinogens as Mutagens in the Salmonella/Microsome Test: Assay of 300 Chemicals: Discussion. *Proc. Natl. Acad. Sciences* 73:950, 1976.
McConnell, J. The Changing Nature of Science and Technology and Its Implica-

tions for Managing Health Delivery Organizations. In Abernathy, W. et al. (Eds.), *The Management of Health Care*. Cambridge, Mass.: Ballinger Publishing Company, 1974.

McDermott, W. Evaluating the Physician and His Technology. *Daedalus* 106:135, 1977.

McKeown, T. *The Role of Medicine, Dream, Mirage, or Nemesis?* London: The Nuffield Provincial Hospitals Trust, 1976.

McKinlay, J. and McKinlay, S. The Questionable Contribution of Medical Measures to the Decline of Mortality in the United States in the Twentieth Century. *MMFQ/Health and Society* 55:405, 1977.

MacMahon, B. et al. *Epidemiologic Methods*. Boston: Little, Brown and Company, 1960.

McNeil, B. Approaches to Efficacy Assessment. Presented at the Meeting on Development and Dissemination of Biomedical Innovations: Foundations for Program Development, Mt. Pocono, Pennsylvania, March 17–19, 1980.

McNeil, B. and Adelstein, S. Evaluation of Diagnostic Screening Tests: A Case Study of Hypertension. In Potchen, E. (Ed.), *Current Concepts in Nuclear Medicine*, Volume 3. St. Louis: The C.V. Mosby Company, 1977.

McNeil, B. and Adelstein, S. Determining the Value of Diagnostic and Screening Tests. *J. Nucl. Med.* 17:439, 1976.

McNeil, B. et al. Rationale for Seeking Occult Metastases in Patients with Bronchogenic Carcinoma *Surgical Gyn. Obstet.* 144:389, 1977.

McPeek, B. et al. The End Result: Quality of Life. In Bunker, J. et al. (Eds.), *Costs, Risks, and Benefits of Surgery*. New York: Oxford University Press, 1977.

McPherson, K. and Fox, M. Treatment of Breast Cancer. In Bunker, J. et al. (Eds.), *Costs, Risks, and Benefits of Surgery*. New York: Oxford University Press, 1977.

Madjid, H. *The Optacon (Optical-to-Tactile Converter)*. A Study for the National Science Foundation. Washington, D.C.: Arthur D. Little, Inc., 1975.

Mahler, H. Health—A Demystification of Medical Technology. *Lancet* 2:829, 1975.

Mahoney, T. *The Merchants of Life*. New York: Harper & Brothers, 1959.

Manley, S. and Ashley, S. AHA Research Capsule No. 24, Sources of Funding for Construction. *Hospitals* 51:59, 1977.

Mansfield, E. *Industrial Research and Technological Innovation: An Econometric Analysis*. New York: W. W. Norton & Co., 1958.

Mansfield, E. et al. *Research and Innovation in the Modern Corporation*. New York: W.W. Norton & Co., 1971.

Marieskind, H. *An Evaluation of Caesarean Section in the United States. Executive Summary*, (Draft). Washington, D.C.: Department of Health, Education, and Welfare, Office of the Assistant Secretary for Planning and Evaluation/Health, June 1979.

Mather, H. et al. Acute Myocardial Infarction: Home and Hospital Treatment. *Br. Med. J.* 3:334, 1971.

Maugh, T. Diabetes Therapy: Can New Techniques Halt Complications? *Science* 190:1281, 1975.

Mausner, J. and Bahn, A. *Epidemiology*. Philadelphia: W.B. Saunders Co., 1974.

Mechanic, D. Approaches to Controlling the Costs of Medical Care: Short-Range and Long-Range Alternatives. *New Eng. J. Med.* 298:249, 1978.

Mechanic, D. The Growth of Medical Technology and Bureaucracy: Implications for Medical Care. *MMFQ/Health and Society* 55:61, 1977.

Mechanic, D. *Politics, Medicine, and Social Science*. New York: John Wiley & Sons, 1974.

Mechanic, D. *Public Expectations and Health Care*. New York: Wiley-Interscience, 1972.

Meier, P. Statistics and Medical Experimentation. *Biometrics* 31:511, 1975.

Mesthene, E. The Role of Technology in Society. In Teich, A. (Ed.), *Technology and Man's Future*. New York: St. Martin's Press, 1977.

Miles, R. *The Department of Health, Education, and Welfare*. New York: Praeger Publishers, 1974.

Morehead, M. Evaluating Quality of Medical Care in the Neighborhood Health Center Program of the Office of Economic Opportunity. *Medical Care* 8:118, 1970.

Morehead, M. et al. Comparisons Between OEO Neighborhood Health Centers and Other Health Care Providers of Ratings of the Quality of Health Care. *Amer. J. Pub. Health* 61:1294, 1971.

Morehead, M. et al. *A Study of the Quality of Hospital Care Secured by a Sample of Teamster Family Members in New York City*. New York: Columbia University School of Public Health and Administrative Medicine, 1964.

Morse, E. et al. Hospital Costs and Quality of Care: An Organizational Perspective. *Milbank Memorial Fund Quarterly* 52:315, 1974.

Moskowitz, M. et al. Lack of Efficacy of Thermography as a Screening Tool for Minimal and Stage I Breast Cancer. *New Eng. J. Med.* 295:249, 1976.

Mushkin, S. *Biomedical Research: Costs and Benefits*. Cambridge, Mass.: Ballinger Publishing Company, 1979.

Mushkin, S. et al. Returns to Biomedical Research 1900-1975: An Initial Assessment of Impacts on Health Expenditures. Washington, D.C.: Public Services Laboratory, Georgetown University, 1976.

National Center for Health Statistics, National Center for Health Services Research. *Health United States. 1979.* DHEW Publication No. (PHS) 80-1232. Hyattsville, Maryland: Department of Health, Education, and Welfare, 1980.

National Center for Health Statistics, National Center for Health Services Research. *Health United States. 1978.* DHEW Publication No. (PHS) 78-1232. Hyattsville, Maryland: Department of Health Education, and Welfare, 1978.

National Heart and Lung Institute. *The Totally Implantable Artificial Heart*. A Report of the Artificial Heart Assessment Panel. Bethesda, Maryland: National Institutes of Health, 1973.

National Institutes of Health. *Consensus Development Conference Summaries,*

1977–1978. Bethesda, Maryland: Department of Health, Education, and Welfare, 1979.
National Institutes of Health. *NIH Inventory of Clinical Trials: Fiscal year 1975*, Volumes I and II. Bethesda, Maryland: Department of Health, Education, and Welfare, 1977a.
National Institutes of Health. *The Responsibilities of NIH at the Health Research/ Health Care Interface*. Draft Report to the Office of the Director. Bethesda, Maryland: Department of Health, Education, and Welfare, February 14, 1977b.
National Institutes of Health. Thirty-Third Meeting, Advisory Committee to the Director, NIH. Briefing Book. Bethesda, Maryland: Department of Health, Education, and Welfare, December 2–3, 1976.
Needleman, J. The Management of Medical Technology in Canada. Draft Paper for the Office of Technology Assessment, Congress of the United States, Washington, D.C., 1979.
Neuhauser, D. and Jonsson, E. Managerial Response to New Health Care Technology: Coronary Artery Bypass Surgery. In Abernathy, W.J. et al. (Eds.), *The Management of Health Care*. Cambridge, Mass.: Ballinger Publishing Co., 1974.
Neuhauser, D. and Lewicki, A. National Health Insurance and the Sixth Stool Guaiac. *Policy Analysis* 2:175, 1976.
Neutra, R. et al. The Effects of Fetal Monitoring on Neonatal Death Rates. *New Eng. J. Med.* 299:324, 1978.
Newsholme, A. *Evolution of Preventive Medicine*. Baltimore, Maryland: The Williams & Wilkins Company, 1927.
Nitzkin, J. Rubella Vaccination Policies. *New Eng. J. Med.* 294:1126, 1976.
Noll, R. The Consequences of Public Utility Regulation of Hospitals. In *Controls on Health Care*, Papers of the Conference on Regulation in the Health Industry, January 7–9, 1974. Washington, D.C.: National Academy of Sciences, 1975.
Oakes, J. Clinical Engineering—The Problems and the Promise. *Science* 190:239, 1975.
Office of the Assistant Secretary for Health. NCHCT Fact Sheet. Washington, D.C.: Department of Health, Education, and Welfare, n.d.
Office of Health Economics. *Renal Failure: A Priority in Health?* London. April, 1978, pp. 31–32.
Office of Planning, Evaluation, and Legislation, Health Services Administration. *PSRO: An Evaluation of the Professional Standards Review Organizations. Volume 1: Executive Summary*. Report No. (OPEL) 77–12. Washington, D.C.: Department of Health, Education, and Welfare, 1977.
Office of Technology Assessment. *Policy Implications of the Computed Tomography (CT) Scanner: An Up-Date* (Draft). Washington, D.C., 1980.
Office of Technology Assessment. *Changes in the Future Use and Characteristics of the Automobile Transportation System*. Publication No. OTA–T–83. Washington, D.C.: GPO, 1979a.

Office of Technology Assessment. *Nutrition Research Alternatives*. Publication No. OTA–F–74. Washington, D.C.: GPO, 1979b.
Office of Technology Assessment. *A Review of Selected Federal Vaccine and Immunization Policies*. Publication No. OTA–H–96. Washington, D.C.: GPO, 1979c.
Office of Technology Assessment. *Assessing the Efficacy and Safety of Medical Technologies*. Publication No. OTA–H–75. Washington, D.C.: GPO, 1978a.
Office of Technology Assessment. *Policy Implications of the Computed Tomography (CT) Scanner*. Publication No. OTA–H–56. Washington, D.C.: GPO, 1978b.
Office of Technology Assessment. *Cancer Testing Technology and Saccharin*. Publication No. OTA–H–55. Washington, D.C.: GPO, 1977.
Office of Technology Assessment. *Development of Medical Technology: Opportunities for Assessment*. Publication No. OTA–H–34. Washington, D.C.: GPO, 1976.
Omenn, G. and Ball, J. The Role of Health Technology Evaluation, A Policy Perspective. In Proceedings of Conference on Health Care Technology Evaluation. Columbia, Missouri. November 6–7, 1978.
Peltzman, S. *Regulation of Pharmaceutical Innovation: The 1962 Amendments*. Washington, D.C.: American Enterprise Institute for Public Policy Research, 1974.
Pennell, M. and Stewart, P. *State Licensing of Health Occupations*. Washington, D.C.: Department of Health, Education, and Welfare, 1968.
Perrott, G. The Federal Employees Health Benefits Program. Washington, D.C.: Department of Health, Education, and Welfare, 1971.
Perrow, C. Hospitals: Technology, Structure, and Goals. In March, J. (Ed.), *Handbook of Organizations*. Chicago: Rand McNally, 1965. Quoted in Committee on Technology and Health Care, *Medical Technology and the Health Care System*. Washington, D.C.: National Academy of Sciences, 1979, p. 26.
Peterson, O. et al. An Analytical Study of North Carolina General Practice. *J. Med. Ed. 31*, (Part 2), December, 1956.
Pineault, R. The Effect of Medical Training Factors on Physician Utilization Behavior. *Medical Care 15*:51, 1977.
Pineault, R. The Effect of Prepaid Group Practice on Physicians' Utilization Behavior. *Medical Care 14*:121, 1976.
Policy Research, Inc. *The Final Report: A Comprehensive Study of the Ethical, Legal, and Social Implications of Advances in Biomedical and Behavioral Research and Technology*. Prepared for the National Commission for the Protection of Human Subjects of Biomedical and Behavioral Research, Bethesda, Maryland, 1977.
Prahalad, C. and Abernathy, W. A Strategy Approach to the Management of Technology in the Health System. In Abernathy, W. et al. (Eds.), *The Management of Health Care*. Cambridge, Mass.: Ballinger Publishing Company, 1974.
President's Biomedical Research Panel. *Report*. DHEW Publication Number (OS) 76–500. Washington, D.C.: GPO, 1976.

Prest, A. and Turvey, R. Cost Benefit Analysis: A Survey. *Econ. J.* 75:683, 1965.
Preston, T. *Coronary Artery Surgery: A Critical Review.* New York: Raven Press, 1977.
Public Health Service. *Forward Plan for Health, FY 1977–81.* DHEW Publication No. (OS) 76–50024. Washington, D.C.: Department of Health, Education, and Welfare, 1975.
Putnam, S. and Banta, D. The Consumer and Primary Care. In Noble, J. (Ed.), *Primary Care and the Practice of Medicine.* Boston: Little, Brown and Company, 1976.
Randal, J. Is Fetal Monitoring Safe? Widely Used Technique Needs More Testing. *The Washington Post,* Sunday, April 16, 1978, p. B3.
Rapoport, J. Diffusion of Technological Innovation Among Non-Profit Firms: A Case Study of Radioisotopes in U.S. Hospitals. *J. Econ. Business* 30:108, 1978.
Redisch, M. Hospital Inflationary Mechanisms. Presented at the Meeting of the Western Economic Association, Las Vegas, Nevada, June 10–12, 1974.
Reich, W. (Ed.). *Encyclopedia of Bioethics.* New York: The Free Press, 1978.
Reidel, D. et al. *Federal Employees Health Benefit Program Utilization Study.* Rockville, Maryland: National Center for Health Services Research, Department of Health, Education, and Welfare, 1975.
Reinhardt, U. Health Manpower Policy and the Cost of Health Care. Presented at the National Health Leadership Conference, Washington, D.C., June 27–28, 1977.
Reinhardt, U. A Production Function for Physicians Services. *Review Econ. Stat.* 54:55, 1972.
Reiser, S. *Medicine and the Reign of Technology.* New York: Cambridge University Press, 1978.
Rettig, R. *Cancer Crusade.* Princeton, N.J.: Princeton University Press, 1977.
Rettig, R. End-Stage Renal Disease and the "Cost" of Medical Technology. In Altman, S. and Blendon, R. (Eds.), *Medical Technologies—The Culprit Behind Health Care Costs?* DHEW Publication No. (PHS) 79–3216. Hyattsville, Maryland: National Center for Health Services Research and Bureau of Health Planning, 1979a.
Rettig, R. Implementing the End-Stage Renal Disease Program of Medicare. Draft Report for the Health Care Financing Administration, Washington, D.C., July 1979b.
Rettig, R. The Role of Formal Analysis in Federal Policy Formulation Toward End-Stage Renal Disease. Draft Paper for the Office of Technology Assessment, Congress of the United States, Washington, D.C., 1979c.
Rettig, R. et al. *Criteria for the Allocation of Resources to Research and Development: A Review of the Literature.* Washington, D.C.: National Science Foundation, 1974.
Richardson, W. et al. *The Seattle Prepaid Health Care Project: Comparison of Health Services Delivery.* Seattle: University of Washington, 1977.
Roemer, M. The Influence of Prepaid Physician's Service on Hospital Utilization. *Hospitals* 32:48, 1958.

Roemer, M. and Shain, M. *Hospital Utilization Under Insurance*. Chicago: American Hospital Association, 1959.

Roemer, M. and Shonick, W. HMO Performance. *Milbank Memorial Fund Quarterly* 51:271, 1973.

Rogers, E. and Shoemaker, F. *Communication of Innovations, A Cross Cultural Approach*. New York: The Free Press, 1971.

Rosen, G. Preventive Medicine in the United States, 1900–1975. In *Preventive Medicine, USA*, Task Force Reports Sponsored by The John E. Fogarty International Center for Advanced Study in the Health Sciences and the American College of Preventive Medicine. New York: Prodist, 1976.

Rosen, G. The Hospital: Historical Sociology of a Community Institution. In Friedson, E. (Ed.), *The Hospital in Modern Society*. New York: The Free Press, 1963.

Rosenthal, G. Anticipating the Costs and Benefits of New Technology: A Typology for Policy. In Altman, S. and Blendon, R. (Eds.), *Medical Technology: The Culprit Behind Health Care Costs?* DHEW Publication No. (PHS) 79–3216. Hyattsville, Maryland: National Center for Health Service Research and Bureau of Health Planning, 1979.

Russell, L. *Technology in Hospitals: Medical Advances and Their Diffusion*. Washington, D.C.: The Brookings Institution, 1979.

Russell, L. How Much Does Medical Technology Cost? *Bull. New York Acad. Med.* 54:124, 1978.

Russell, L. The Diffusion of New Hospital Technologies in the United States. *Intl. J. Health Services* 6:557, 1976.

Russell, L. and Burke, C. *Technological Diffusion in the Hospital Sector*. Washington, D.C.: National Planning Association, 1975.

Rutstein, D. et al. Measuring the Quality of Medical Care: A Clinical Method. *New Eng. J. Med.* 294:582, 1976.

Salkever, D. and Bice, T. *Hospital Certificate-of-Need Controls: Impact on Investment, Costs and Use*. Washington, D.C.: American Enterprise Institute for Public Policy Research, 1979.

Salkever, D., and Bice, T. The Impact of Certificate-of-Need Controls on Hospital Investment. *MMFQ/Health and Society* 54:185, 1976.

Sax, S. International Project on Health Care Systems and Medical Technology, Description of Australian Systems. Draft Paper for the Office of Technology Assessment, Congress of the United States, Washington, D.C., 1979.

Schelling, T. The Life You Save May Be Your Own. In Chase, S. (Ed.), *Problems in Public Expenditure Analysis*. Washington, D.C.: The Brookings Institution, 1968.

Schifrin, L. Personal Communication. March, 1980.

Schifrin, L. and Tayan, J. The Drug Lag: An Interpretative Review of the Literature. *Intl. J. Health Services* 7:359, 1977.

Schnee, J. and Caglarcan, E. Economic Structure and Performance of the Ethical Pharmaceutical Industry. In Lindsay, C.M. (Ed.), *The Pharmaceutical Industry*. New York: John Wiley & Sons, 1978.

Schoenbaum, S. et al. Benefit-Cost Analysis of Rubella Vaccination Policy. *New Eng. J. Med.* 294:306, 1976a.

Schoenbaum, S. et al. The Swine Influenza Decision. *New Eng. J. Med.* 295:759, 1976b.

Schor, S. and Karten, I. Statistical Evaluation of Medical Journal Manuscripts. *JAMA* 195:145, 1966.

Schroeder, S. and Showstack, J. The Dynamics of Medical Technology Use: Analysis and Policy Options. In Altman, S. and Blendon, R. (Eds.), *Medical Technology: The Culprit Behind Health Care Costs?* DHEW Publication No. (PHS) 79–3216. Hyattsville, Maryland: National Center for Health Services and Bureau of Health Planning, 1979.

Schroeder, S. and Showstack, J. Financial Incentives to Perform Medical Procedures and Laboratory Tests: Illustrative Models of Office Practice. *Medical Care* 16:289, 1978.

Schroeder, S. et al. Use of Laboratory Tests and Pharmaceuticals. *JAMA* 225:969, 1973.

Schultze, C. *The Public Use of the Private Interest.* Washington, D.C.: The Brookings Institution, 1977.

Schweitzer, S. and Luce, B. *A Cost-Effective Approach to Cervical Cancer Detection.* Report to National Center for Health Services Research, Department of Health, Education, and Welfare, Washington, D.C., 1978.

Scitovsky, A. Changes in the Use of Ancillary Services for Common Illness. In Altman, S. and Blendon, R. (Eds.), *Medical Technology: The Culprit Behind Health Care Costs?* DHEW Publication No. (PHS) 79–3216. Hyattsville, Maryland: National Center for Health Services Research and Bureau of Health Planning, 1979.

Scitovsky, A. Changes in the Costs of Treatment of Selected Illnesses, 1951–65. *Amer. Econ. Review* 53:1182, 1967.

Scitovsky, A. and McCall, N. Changes in the Cost of Treatment of Selected Illnesses, 1951–1964–1971. DHEW Publication No. (HRA) 77–361. Washington, D.C.: National Center for Health Services Research, 1976.

Seeff, L. et al. A Randomized, Double Blind Controlled Trial of the Efficacy of Immune Serum Globulin for the Prevention of Post-Transfusion Hepatitis. *Gastroenterology* 72:111, 1977.

Senate. *Report. Clinical Laboratory Improvement Act of 1977.* Report No. 95–360. Washington, D.C.: Congress of the United States, 1977.

Sencer, D. and Axnick, N. Utilization of Cost/Benefit Analysis in Planning Prevention Programs. *Acta Med. Scand.* 576:(Suppl.):123, 1975.

Shapiro, S. Medical Care: Issues of Evaluation. *Science* 199:964, 1978.

Shapiro, S. Evidence on Screening for Breast Cancer from a Randomized Trial. *Cancer* 39:2772, 1977.

Shapiro, S. End Result Measurements of Quality of Medical Care. *Milbank Memorial Fund Quarterly* 45:7, 1967.

Shapiro, S. et al. Periodic Breast Cancer Screening in Reducing Mortality from Breast Cancer. *JAMA* 215:1777, 1971.

Shapiro, S. et al. Further Observations on Prematurity and Perinatal Mortality in a General Population and in the Population of a Prepaid Group Practice Medical Care Plan. *Amer. J. Pub. Health* 50:1304, 1960.

Shortell, S. et al. The Effects of Management Practices on Hospital Efficiency and Quality of Care. In Shortell, S. and Brown, M. (Eds.), *Organizational Research in Hospitals*. Chicago: Blue Cross Association, 1976.

Showstack, J. and Schroeder, S. The Cost-Effectiveness of Upper Gastrointestinal Endoscopy. Draft Paper for the Office of Technology Assessment, Congress of the United States, Washington, D.C., 1979.

Showstack, J. et al. Fee-for-Service Physician Payment: Analysis of Current Methods and Their Development. *Inquiry* 16:230, 1979.

Shryock, R.H. *The Development of Modern Medicine*. New York: Hafner Publishing Co., 1969.

Sigerist, H. *Man and Medicine*. College Park, Maryland: McGrath Publishing Company, 1970 (Copyright 1932).

Silverman, M. and Lee, P. *Pills, Profits, and Politics*. Berkeley, California: University of California Press, 1974.

Silverman, W. The Lesson of Retrolental Fibroplasis. *Scientific American* 236:100, 1977.

Smith, D. and Kaluzny, A. *The White Labyrinth*. Berkeley, California: McCutchan Publishing Corporation, 1975.

Smits, H. The Technology Problem: The Federal Perspective. Presented at the Meeting of the American Public Health Association, New York, November 7, 1979.

Spingarn, N. *Heartbeat: The Politics of Health Research*. Washington, D.C.: Robert B. Luce, Inc., 1976.

Spri. *International Workshop on Evaluation of Medical Technology*. Stockholm, Sweden: Swedish Planning and Rationalization Institute of the Health Services, 1979.

Stein, J. Riding Herd on Medical Gadgetry. *National Journal* 11:958, 1979.

Stein, J. *Making Medical Choices: Who Is Responsible?* Boston: Houghton Mifflin Company, 1978.

Stevens, R. *American Medicine and the Public Interest*. New Haven, Conn.: Yale University Press, 1971.

Stocking, B. The Management of Medical Technology in the U.K. Draft Paper for the Office of Technology Assessment, Congress of the United States, Washington, D.C., 1979.

Stocking, B. *The Image and the Reality: A Case Study of the Impacts of Medical Technology*. London: Nuffield Provincial Hospitals Trust, 1978.

Strange, P. and Sumner, A. Predicting Treatment Costs and Life Expectancy for End-Stage Renal Disease. *New Eng. J. Med.* 298:372, 1978.

Strickland, S. *Politics, Science & Dread Disease*. Cambridge, Mass.: Harvard University Press, 1972.

Sullivan, J. Priest in Coma Case Calls Legal Issue More Difficult Than the Moral. *The New York Times*, September 26, 1975, p. 37.

Sun Valley Forum on National Health. Medical Cure and Medical Care. Summary. *Milbank Memorial Fund Quarterly* 50:231, 1972.

Swazey, J. and Fox, R. The Clinical Moratorium. In Fox, R., *Essays in Medical Sociology: Journeys into the Field*. New York: John Wiley & Sons, Inc., 1979.

Takaro, T. et al. The VA Cooperative Randomized Study of Surgery for Coronary Arterial Occlusive Disease. II. Subgroup with Significant Left Main Lesions. *Circulation* 54(Suppl. 3):107, 1976.

Tancredi, L. The Ethics Quagmire and Random Clinical Trials. *Inquiry* 12:171, 1975.

Tannon, C. and Rogers, E. Diffusion Research Methodology: Focus on Health Care Organizations. In Gordon, G. and Fisher, L. (Eds.), *The Diffusion of Medical Technology*. Cambridge, Mass.: Ballinger Publishing Co., 1975.

Thomas, K. *Religion and the Decline of Magic*. New York: Charles Scribner & Sons, 1971.

Thomas, L. *The Lives of a Cell*. New York: The Viking Press, 1974.

Trussell, R. et al. *The Quantity, Quality and Costs of Medical Care Secured by a Sample of Teamster Families in the New York Area*. New York: Columbia University School of Public Health and Administrative Medicine, 1962.

Turney-High, H. *Man and System*. New York: Appleton-Century-Crofts, 1968.

Utterback, J. Innovation in Industry and the Diffusion of Technology. *Science* 183:620, 1976.

Veatch, R. and Branson, R. *Ethics and Health Policy*. Cambridge, Mass.: Ballinger Publishing Company, 1976.

Vecchio, T. Predictive Value of a Single Diagnostic Test in Unselected Populations. *New Eng. J. Med.* 274:1171, 1966.

Visscher, M. *Ethical Constraints and Imperatives in Medical Research*. Springfield, Ill.: Charles C Thomas, Publisher, 1975.

Wagner, E. et al. Influence of Training and Experience in Selecting Criteria to Evaluate Medical Care. *New Eng. J. Med.* 294:871, 1976.

Wagner, J. The Feasibility of Economic Evaluation of Diagnostic Procedures: The Case of CT Scanning. Draft paper for the Office of Technology Assessment, Congress of the United States, Washington, D.C., 1979.

Wagner, J. A Study of the Impact of Hospital Reimbursement Policy on the Diffusion of New Medical Technology. Project Proposal Funded by the Health Care Financing Administration, Grant No. 18–P–97113/3–01, 1978.

Waitzkin, H. A Marxian Interpretation of the Growth and Development of Coronary Care Technology. *Amer. J. Pub. Health* 69:1260, 1979.

Waldman, S. The Effect of Changing Technology on Hospital Costs. *Social Security Administration Research and Statistics Note, No. 4*. DHEW Publication No. (SSA) 72–11701. Washington, D.C.: GPO, 1972.

Wan, T. and Livieratos, B. Interpreting a General Index of Subjective Well-Being. *MMFQ/Health and Society* 56:187, 1978.

Wardell, W. and Lasagna, L. *Regulation and Drug Development*. Washington, D.C.: American Enterprise Institute, 1975.

Warner, K. Effects of Hospital Cost Containment on the Development and Use of Medical Technology. *MMFQ/Health and Society* 56:187, 1978.

Warner, K. Treatment Decision Making in Catastrophic Illness. *Medical Care* 25:19, 1977.

Warner, K. A 'Desperation-Reaction' Model of Medical Diffusion. *Health Services Research* 10:369, 1975.

Warner, K. The Need for Some Innovative Concepts of Innovation: An Examination of Research on the Diffusion of Innovations. *Policy Sciences* 5:433, 1974.

Warner, K. et al. *Cost-Benefit and Cost-Effectiveness Analysis in Health Care: Methodology and Literature Review*. Draft Report for the Office of Technology Assessment, Congress of the United States, Washington, D.C., 1979.

Waters, W. A Randomized Controlled Clinical Trial of Ergotamine Tartrate. *Br. J. Soc. Prevent. Med.* 24:65, 1970.

Weil, P. Comparative Costs of the Medicare Program of Seven Prepaid Group Practices and Controls. *MMFQ/Health and Society* 54:339, 1976.

Weinstein, M. Economic Evaluation of Medical Procedures and Technologies: Progress, Problems, and Prospects. In Wagner, J. (Ed.), *Medical Technology*. DHEW Publication No. (PHS) 79-3254. Hyattsville, Maryland: National Center for Health Services Research, 1979.

Weinstein, M. and Stason, W. Foundations of Cost-Effectiveness Analysis for Health and Medical Practices. *New Eng. J. Med.* 296:716, 1977.

Weinstein, M. and Stason, W. *Hypertension: A Policy Perspective*. Cambridge, Mass.: Harvard University Press, 1976.

Weisbrod, B. *Economics of Public Health*. Philadelphia: University of Pennsylvania Press, 1961.

Wennberg, J. and Gittelsohn, A. Health Care Delivery in Maine: I. Patterns of Use of Common Surgical Procedures. *Maine Med. Assoc.* 66:123, 1975.

Wennberg, J. and Gittelsohn, A. Small Area Variations in Health Care Delivery. *Science* 182:1102, 1973.

Whalan, D. The Ethics and Morality of Clinical Trials in Man. *Med. J. Australia* 1:491, 1975.

White, K. Opportunities and Needs for Epidemiology and Health Statistics in the United States. Presented at the Invitational Conference on Epidemiology as the Fundamental Basis for Planning, Administration and Evaluation of Health Services, Baltimore, Maryland, March 2-4, 1975.

White, K. Contemporary Epidemiology. *Intl. J. Epidem.* 3:295, 1974.

White, K. International Comparisons of Health Services Systems. *Milbank Memorial Fund Quarterly* 46:117, 1968. (In 1979, Dr. White stated in a personal communication that he did not believe that the situation had improved.)

White, K. et al. Technology and Health Care. *New Eng. J. Med.* 287:1223, 1972.

Willems, J. Cost-Effectiveness Analysis of Medical Technologies as an Aid to Policymakers. In Goldman, J. (Ed.), *Health Care Technology Evaluation*. Lecture Notes in Medical Informatics, Vol. 6. New York: Springer-Verlag, 1979a.

Willems, J. The Relationship Between the Diffusion of Medical Technology and the Organization and Economics of Health Care Delivery. In Wagner, J. (Ed.), *Medical Technology*. DHEW Publication No. (PHS) 79–3254. Hyattsville, Maryland: National Center for Health Services Research, 1979b.

Willems, J. Linking Third-Party Payment with Prior Technology Evaluation: The Usefulness of Formal Techniques. Presented at the Meeting of the American Public Health Association, New York, November 7, 1979c.

Willems, J. Institutional Methods of Delivering Health Care: Comparative Costs. Unpublished Doctoral Thesis, Montreal, McGill University, 1976.

Willems, J. et al. The Computed Tomography Scanner. In Altman, S. and Blendon, R. (Eds.), *Medical Technology: The Culprit Behind Health Care Costs?* DHEW Publication No. (PHS) 79–3216. Hyattsville, Maryland: National Center for Health Services Research and Bureau of Health Planning, 1979.

Willems, J. et al. Cost-Effectiveness Analysis of Vaccination Against Pneumococcal Pneumonia. *New Eng. J. Med. 303*:553, 1980.

Williams, R. and Hawes, W. Cesarean Section, Fetal Monitoring, and Perinatal Mortality in California. *Amer. J. Pub. Health* 69:864, 1979.

Williamson, J. *Assessing and Improving Health Care Outcomes: The Health Accounting Approach to Quality Assurance*. Cambridge, Mass.: Ballinger Publishing Company, 1978.

Williamson, J. Correctable Deficiencies in Contemporary Quality Assurance. In Williamson, J., *Improving Medical Practice and Health Care*. Cambridge, Mass.: Ballinger Publishing Company, 1977.

Wilson, H. *The American Ideology: Science, Technology and Organization as Modes of Rationality in Advanced Industrial Societies*. London: Routledge & Kegan Paul, 1977.

Wooldridge, D. (Chairman). *Biomedical Science and Its Administration: A Study of the National Institutes of Health*. Report to the President by the NIH Study Committee. Washington, D.C.: GPO, 1965.

Work Group XII. Human Experimentation in Digestive Disease Research. *Gastroenterology* 69:1165, 1975.

World Health Organization. *Long Term Effects of Coronary Bypass Surgery*. Report of a Working Group, The Hague, November, 1977. Copenhagen, Denmark: World Health Organization Regional Office for Europe, 1978.

World Health Organization. *Statistical Indicators for the Planning and Evaluation of Public Health Programmes. Fourteenth Report of the WHO Expert Committee on Health Statistics*. World Health Organization Technical Report Series, No. 472. Geneva, Switzerland, 1971.

Wortman, P. and Rogers, J. Evaluating Health Care Technology. An Example from Electrocardiography. *Evaluation and the Health Professions* 1:3, 1978.

Young, D. Communicating the Findings from Clinical Trials. (Manuscript.) Washington, D.C.: Veterans Administration Scholars Program, 1980.

Index

Accreditation, 162
Actual adopters, 53–54
Adopters, 60–62
Adoption, factors influencing, 58–66
  adopter organization or individual, 60–62
  environment, 62–66
  technology, 58–60
Adoption, federal activities to influence, 66–73
  acquiring specific technologies, 67–68
  financing programs, 71–72
  health planning and reimbursement, 73
  health planning program, 68–71
  promotion of technology, 67
Alcohol, Drug Abuse and Mental Health Administration (ADAMHA), 114
American College of Physicians, Medical Practice Committee (1976), 115
Anatomy and physiology, 22–23
Applied research and development, 39–41
  and clinical testing, 44
  compared to basic research, 40, 42–44
  diagnostic tools, 41
  funding, 48
  goal-orientation, 41
  vitality of, 40
Australia
  fee mechanism, 179
  health planning, 178

  health services research, 176
  national advisory panel on applications and costs of technology, 176

Bacteriology, development of, 25–26
Basic research, 37–39
  compared to applied research, 40, 42–44
  funding, 48
  investigator-initiated research, 51
  medical advances, 39
Bench to bedside lag, 11
Benefit-cost analysis, 128–135
  analyses for policy purposes, 133–134
  compared to cost-effectiveness analysis, 134–135
  limitations, 129–133
  quality of life, 129
  years of life, 129
Bioengineering, 32
Bioethics, 138
Biology
  compared to physical sciences, 42
  development of, 37–38
Blue Cross and Blue Shield
  conformity with planning procedure, 73
  CT scanners, 143–144
  Medical Necessity Program, 197–198
  reimbursement and efficacy, 72
Breast Cancer Detection Demonstration Project (BCDDP), 113
Bureaucratization and technology, 85–86

237

Bureaucratization (cont.)
  bureaucratic functioning, 85–86
  economic efficiency, 86
  loss of caring, 86
  theoretical advantages, 86

Canada
  health planning, 178
  hospital budgeting system, 180
  national health insurance, 88–89
  outpatient care, 179
Capital availability, 64–65
  access to funds, 64
  debt financing, 65
  depreciation, 65
  replacement cost basis, 65
  terms of funding, 64
  See also Financing methods
Capitation payment method, 84
Cardiac pacemaker, 7, 8, 32, 55
Cartesian thought, 22, 24, 28–29
Centers for Disease Control (COC), 68, 133
Certification, 162
Chemistry, history of, 24–25
Chemotherapy for leukemia, 54, 56
Chronic diseases, 12–14
Clinical laboratory, automation of, 75–76
Clinical testing and applied research, 44
Clinical trials, controlled, 106–107, 141–142
  expenditures (1975), 107
  control group, 106
  randomized controlled trials, 107
Committee on the Costs of Medical Care, 158
Computed tomography (CT) scanner, 28, 181–184
  Blue Cross/Blue Shield, 143–144
  controls over, 182–184
  efficacy, 71
  numbers, 182, 183
  operating expenses, 70
  profits from, 64
  purchase of, 62
  social implications, 147
  technology characteristics, 59–60
CON laws, see State certificate-of-need (CON) laws
Coronary bypass surgery, 186–187
Cost-effectiveness analysis, 128–135
  analyses for policy purposes, 133–134
  compared to benefit-cost analysis, 134–135
  cost-effectiveness ratio, 128
  discounting, 131
  limitations, 129–133
  National Center for Health Services Research, 131
  quality-adjusted life years, 129

Descartes, Rene, 22, 24
Desperation-reaction model, 55
Device, 5, 46–47
Diagnostic technology, 5
Diffusion, 53–57
Discounting, 131
Disease, classification of, 23
Drug, 5, 45–46
Drug industry, 31–32
Drug industry products promotion, 81–83
  drug detail men and women, 82
  equipment manufacturer representatives, 82
  expenditures, 82

Economic Stabilization Program, 88
Effectiveness, 98
Efficacy, 94–98
  benefit, 94–96
  and conditions of use, 97–98
  defined, 94, 95, 98
  diagnostic technology benefit, 96
  medical conditions, 96–97
  population affected, 97
  See also Safety
Efficacy and safety, assessment system, 115–121, 193–195

Index

development of information, 195
dissemination, 116, 120–121
effective distribution, 120
identification, 115, 117–119
synthesis, 115, 120
testing, 115, 119–120
Efficacy and safety data, use and users of, 100–101, 102–103
private sector activities, 114–115
Efficacy and safety, estimating of, 101–108
Efficacy and safety information, status of, 121–122
Efficacy and safety relationship, 99–100
England
controlled clinical trials, 175
health planning, 178
National Health Service budgeting, 180
physician consensus, 176
regulation, 177
Environmental factors in technological adoption, 62–66
Epidemiology, 105–106
Ethics, 137–138
Evaluation of specific technologies, 127–135
analyses for policy purposes, 133–134
criteria for coverage, 72
limitations, 129–133
methodology, 128–129
process, 140–143
and social values, 140–143
status of information, 134–135
Experimental Medical Care Review Organization (EMCRO) program, 163–164

Federal funding
historical view, 32–33
research and development, 48–51
ultrasonic imaging, 47
See also Funding
Federal Health Resources Sharing Committee, 68
Fee-for-service, 63, 88

Fee mechanism, 179
Financial costs of medical technology, 18–19
See also Medical expenditures
Financing methods, 63–64
fee-for-service, 63, 88
health insurance, 63
prospective reimbursement, 64, 87–88, 199
third-party payment, 63, 64, 89–91, 197–198
See also Capital availability
Financing use of technology, 197–200
Food and Drug Administration, 20, 109–110, 195–196
classification system, 110–111
medical devices, 110–111
prescription drugs, 109–110
safety and efficacy, 110
Food, Drug and Cosmetic Act (1938), 109
Formal synthesis, 107–108
France
cost-effectiveness analysis, 175
device assessment, 177
drug standards, 177
health planning, 177–178
research and development, 174
Funding for research and development, 47–51

Halfway technology, 12, 27, 124, 192
Health accounting, 170
Health and illness, 139
Health Care Financing Administration (HCFA), 71–72, 73
Health Maintenance Organizations (HMOs), 69, 84, 199
Health planning and reimbursement, 73
Health Planning Program, 68–71
capital investment regulation, 69–71
program deficiencies, 71
Health Standards and Quality Bureau (HSQB), 168

Health Systems Agency (HSA), 69
Hill-Burton program, 65, 67
History
  medical science, 22–23
  medical technology, 14–15, 21–35
  modern developments, 27–28
  therapy, 23–24
Hospital medical staff review committees, 162–163
Hospitals, June 1, 1979, on medical technology, 82
Hospitals and technology, 83–84

Immunization Practice Advisory Committee (IPAC), 67–68
Informal evaluation, 104–105
Intensive care units, 54
Interventionist technology, 132

Joint Commission on Accreditation of Hospitals (JCAH), 162

Leucotomy, 56, 121
  in England and Wales, 57
Licensing, 159, 161–162
  institutional licensure, 161–162
  medical licensure, 161

Magic bullet, 27
Malpractice liability, 81
  defensive medicine, 81
  fear of malpractice, 81, 143, 189
Market structure, 65–66
  physician-population ratio, 66
Medicaid, 31, 33, 71, 72, 84, 90–91
Medical care, organization of, 30, 83–86, 192–193
  bureaucratization, 85–86
  financing of, 31
  hospitals, 83–84
  medical practice, 84–85
Medical care, quality of, *see* Quality assurance
Medical Device Amendments (1976), 110
Medical device regulation, U.S., 177

Medical education, 29–30, 192
Medical expenditures and role of technology, 124–127
  national costs, 1978, 123
  systemwide effect, 127
  technology as a residual, 124
Medical instruments, 24
Medical practice and technology, 84–85
  capitation, 84
  Health Maintenance Organizations, 84
  practice settings, 84–85
Medical specialization, 78–80
  excess supply of physicians, 79
  improved quality of care, 78–79
  learning curve, 80
  medical education, 79
  use of technologies, 80
Medical technology, 4–7
  benefits, 11–17
  communication about, 58
  federal reactions, 20
  financial costs, 18–19
  history, 14–15, 21–35
  risks, 17–18
  social impacts, 19–20
Medical technology evaluation, historical review, 33–35
Medicare, 31, 33, 71, 72, 84, 90–91, 163, 200
Mortality rates
  England and Wales, 14–16
  U.S., 12, 13
Multiple Risk Factor Intervention Trials (MRFIT), 107

National Blood Pressure Education Program, 67
National Center for Health Care Technology (NCHCT), 72, 108–109, 134, 155, 196
  functions, 108
  Medicare recommendations, 108
  National Council, 109
National Center for Health Services Research, 131, 155

Index

National Guidelines for Health Planning, 1978, 70
National Health Planning and Resources Development Act, 69
  1974, 69, 70, 155
  1979 amendment, 69, 71
National Institutes of Health (NIH), 20, 111–113
  Associate Director of Medical Applications of Research, 113
  clinical trial support, 111–112
  consensus development, 112–113
  formation of, 33
  institutes' names, 111
  mission, 111
  orientation, 190
National Research Act 1974, 140
National Science Foundation (NSF), 155
Netherlands, 177

Office of Technology Assessment (OTA), 134, 154–155
  Health Program reports, 203–208
Organization, *see* Medical care organization

Patient needs and technology, 76
Patients' rights, 141
Payment methods, 87–89
  capitation, 88
  cross-subsidization. 87
  fee-for-service, 63, 88
  fee scale, 87
  hospital charge structures, 87
  prospective reimbursement, 64, 87–88, 199
Penicillin, 27, 31
Pharmaceutical Manufacturers Association, 82–83
Pharmacology, 26–27, 31–32
Physician and technology, 77–80
Policies toward medical technology, 187–188

Policy research, *see* Technology Assessment
Potential adopters, 53–54
Preclinical tests, 101–104
Priorities, setting of, 193
Private sector organizations
  dealing with efficacy data, 114–115
  dealing with social implications, 155
  and funding for research, 48, 50
Procedure, 5, 47
Professionalism, 77–78
Professional Standards Review Organizations (PSROs), 20, 81, 163–168
  development, 164–167
  EMCRO program, 163–164
  Professional Standards Review Council, 165
  shortcomings, 167–168
Prospective reimbursement, 64, 87–88, 199
Public Law 92–603, 164, 165
Public Law 92–623, 108

Quality assurance, 157–171
  activities and programs, 160–163
  conceptual approaches, 158–160
  current status, 168–171
  PSRO program, 163–168
Quality of care
  defined, 158
  history, 158
  research, 168–171
Quality of care assessment, 159–163

Randomization, *see* Clinical trials
Regional Medical Program (RMP), 67
Regulatory programs, strengthening of, 195–196
Renal dialysis, 19, 184–185
  1972 Social Security Amendment, 32
  policies, 184–185
  Schribner shunt, 32
  third-party coverage, 90
  treatment by country, 185

Research and development, 37–52
  applied research and development, 39–41
  basic research, 37–39
  control of, 191–192
  device development, 46
  drug development, 45–46
  funding, 47–51
  nontraditional research, 44–45
  planning problems, 51–52
  procedures development, 47
Risks of medical technology, 17–18, 98–99

Safety, 98–99
  See also Efficacy and safety
Scientific Apparatus Manufacturers Association, 83
Sequential Multiple-Analyzer (SMA), 32
Sigmoid curve, in diffusion, 53–54
Social impacts, 19–20, 148
Social implications of medical technology, 144–156
Social Security Act, 71
  Section 1122 review, 69, 70
Social values, 137–144
State certificate-of-need (CON) laws, 69, 70, 71, 200

Sulfanilamide, 34
Sweden, 175, 179–181

Technological change, process of, 7–11
Technology, 1–4
Technology Assessment (TA), 151–154
Thalidomide, 17
Third-party payment, 63–64, 89–91, 197, 198
Tracer method, 169–170

United Kingdom, *see* England
U.S. Department of Health and Human Services, Forward Plan for Health, 39–40
U.S. DHEW Health Research Principles, 51

Vertical integration, 61–62
Veterans Administration (VA), 68

West Germany
  drug regulation, 176–177
  health planning, 178
  research and development, 174
World Health Organization, definition of health, 139

X-ray, development of, 25